I0413318

Trigger Point Made Easy

Learn Trigger Point Therapy by Using Body Tools to Apply Pressure to Your Self

Carolyn Gibson
LMT, MI, CE Provider for Texas Massage
Therapist

DEDICATION

This is dedicated to those who are in chronic pain and tension. A big thanks to my clients whose feedback helped me more than any class or lessons. This is dedicated to massage therapist all over who also hurt and have dedicated themselves to relieving the suffering of their clients.

CONTENTS

ACKNOWLEDGMENTS

Although this is meant to be a manual for CE classes for Texas Massage Therapist., this will benefit anyone with chronic pain and tension. If you are a Texas Massage Therapist you can visit my website: www.TexasMassageTherapistCEU.com for information about my classes.

If you are a Massage Therapist instructor or CE provider you can contact me for bulk prices on this manual. 903 833 1024

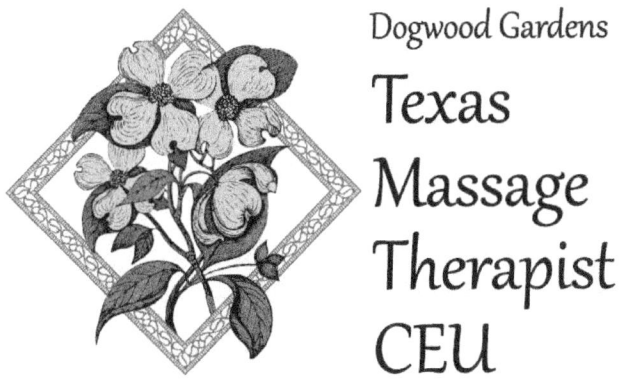

Dogwood Gardens
Texas
Massage
Therapist
CEU

Disclaimer:

This book does not offer medical advice to the reader and is not intended as a replacement for appropriate health care and treatment. Readers should always consult their licensed physician.

1 INTRODUCTION

Learn Trigger Point Therapy by appling pressure with self massager tools to yourself first, to learn, to know and truly feel the Trigger Point Difference. Then you can confidently integrate Trigger Point Therapy into your practice

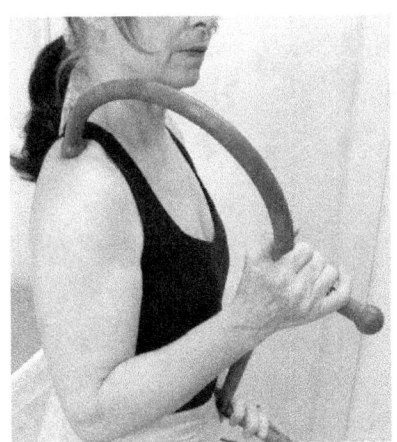 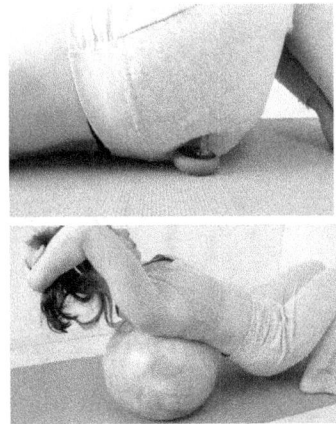

The Thera Cane, The Knobble II, and Ball

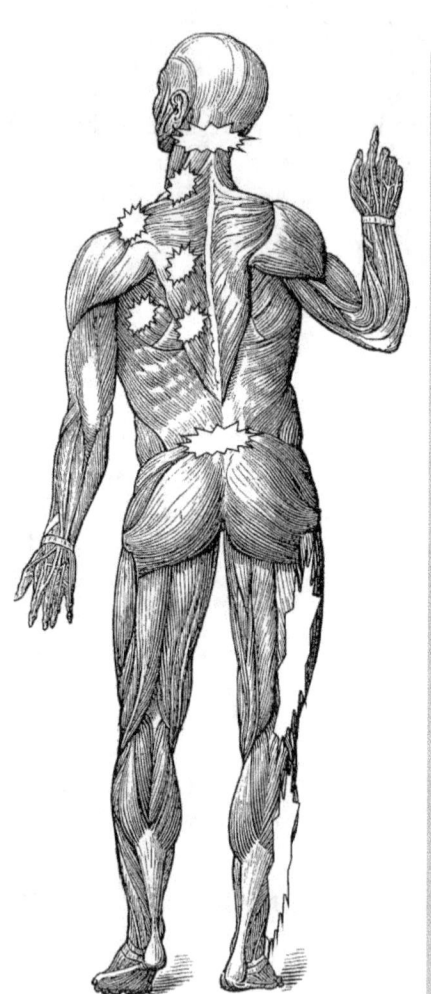

Easy to learn and easy to apply techniques to relieve stress knots and chronic pain in the:

Neck

Headaches caused by neck tension

Shoulder Area

Low Back

Hip and Hip Joints

Sciatica

This class covers these most common complaints of pain and tension that you have and your clients have.

After learning Trigger Point Therapy and studying all the different areas, I soon realized I was treating these same areas in all my clients.

These areas work together and affect each other.

The muscles from the top of your head down, meet at the pelvis. All the muscle from your toes up, meet at the pelvis. Your pelvis is your center of balance. Your body wants to see "eye level". If your pelvis is out of balance, your body will pull and twist various muscles, both above and below the hips, trying to obtain "eye level".

Many times it may be that pain in your bottom causing that pain in your neck and shoulders.

Using these tools on ourselves, we are not only treating our own aches and pains but we are learning the feel of our muscles releasing. We feel how the release of one muscle affects other muscles.

Don't get the wrong idea that you will feel this magic release of all your pain. You may feel some pressure let up, it will be the next day or even the day after that you will feel the big difference.

Because we feel our muscles releasing, we do not just learn, we know.

The difference in learning and knowing is like when we were young and learning what hot means.
You learned from your parents that hot hurts.
When you touched the fire, you knew what hot meant.

You cannot treat all Trigger Points with self treatment. This will not be the only Trigger Point class you will ever need to take. This by no means covers all the Trigger Points. When you are ready to dig deeper, and learn more I encourage you to take Trigger Point classes designed more for treating your clients.

Keep in mind, if you try to learn too much at one time, you will get overwhelmed and then will not know where to begin.

We go into massage therapy because we have compassion and desire to make others feel better and relieve their pain. We are naturally caring people. It hurts us when we are unsuccessful. We may also have gone into massage therapy to find the cure for our own aches and pain. One thing for sure if we did not have aches and pain when we started, we do now. Caring for others has its' price. We can be of no use to others if we ourselves are in pain. Muscle tension kills your joy, creates a negative attitude, and drains your energy.

Self healing or self treatment is the mission of this class. Enjoy this class and have fun. Forget muscle groups and complicated Trigger Point charts, and diagnosing referred pain. This class will use touch and feel anatomy. This class will start with using body tools to locate general Trigger Point areas on your own body. Only when you know how they feel on yourself and you experience the release, can you truly appreciate what your client is feeling and have true confidence in what you are doing. Self treatment will help you understand the amount of pressure to apply. It will develop your healing instinct which will naturally guide you in treating your clients.

I know this body work is effective, I used it on myself after years of constant pain.

I had **the headache**, for over 20 years. It is with me day in and day out. On good days, it was barely there. On ordinary days it was there just enough to drain my energy. I thought, "please, God, don't let it get any worse, I have too much to do." At the end of the day I felt like my head was too heavy for my neck to support.

On bad days it sent me to bed. The only relief was to go to bed and lie flat. I wanted the lights off. I couldn't raise my head to read a book or watch TV. And to top it all off, I really wasn't sleepy enough to sleep through the pain.

It would start at the base of my neck and climb up to the base of my skull.

The pain traveled to my ears and to my teeth. My head hurt all over. There was intense pressure at the base of my skull behind the ear. My shoulders and shoulder blades were tense. I felt if someone would just stick an ice pick in my skull I would feel better.

Pain relievers did absolutely no good.

For years I called it a sinus headache. If it were a sinus headache wouldn't I have sinus congestion? If I wasn't all clogged up, maybe it wasn't a sinus headache.

Self treatment using Trigger Point brought me relief.

Some people may receive relief after the first treatment. For me it took repeated treatments the first week to break the cycle. After the first week, maintenance only took 5-10 minutes a day. After a year it is on as needed basis. Everyone is different and you will develop your own routine.

If you are in a "flare up" on one of those really bad days, this will not stop it that day. But it will prevent it from being there the next day. Your best defense is to use Trigger Point at the first sign of tension.

If it has started because you are totally 'pissed off', it will not work. You will have to let go of the anger first.

Once you relieve yourself of this pain, you realize how heavy pain is. You will feel lighter.

Then I was blessed with sciatica. I say blessed because it must have been God's way of pushing me to find relief for myself so I could help others. I suffered for over 10 years before I discovered self treatment using Trigger Point Therapy.

When I first discovered using body tools to treat myself with Trigger Point Therapy, I received tremendous relief, but not complete relief. I had to treat myself daily to keep the pain and tension at bay. I knew I was missing something. So I continued to dig deeper, researching other methods.

Once I released these Trigger Points, what was I doing to re- activate them?

One was the recliner. Recliners are made for men, or at least someone much taller. Sitting in the recliner pushed my head forward, creating pain and tension in my neck. I bought a 4" cushion to sit on, raising my neck past the curve in the recliner. For you it may as little as a 1 inch or 2 inch cushion if you have the same problem.

Sitting in the church pew created sciatic nerve pain in my hips. I did not need a cushion to raise me up but something to push me forward so that my feet would touch the ground and the bench would not cut off my circulation at the knees. I did not need 4 inches, just 1-2 inches. I stacked the song books behind my back.

Your problem could be worn out heels on your shoes or changing the size of heels you are accustomed to.

Instead of Trigger Point you might need to make some minor modifications in your life.

It wasn't until I started using these other body treatments that I was able to truly break the cycle, making self treatment even more effective.

I discovered deep breathing, body rolling, and body arching.

This class is all about Trigger Point Therapy, and we will cover:

A brief overview of Trigger Point Therapy:

    What is a Trigger Point?

    What causes Trigger Points?

    What does a Trigger Point feel like?

How to apply Trigger Point pressure?

How much pressure to apply?

Why does Trigger Point Therapy work?

Locating and treating Trigger Points:

We will start with the Thera Cane and then go to the Knobble II.

How to use the Thera Cane

Trigger Points Sites for the Neck, Shoulders and Headache caused by Neck Tension using the Thera Cane.

Trigger Point Sites in the front of the body using the Thera Cane and fingers.

The Knobble II:

Low Back Pain, Hips, and Hip Joints, Down the Leg or Sciatica

Body Arching for Low Back Pain

The McKenzie Push Up

Body Rolling

Deep Breathing

Review the importance of long gliding strokes to smooth out the fascia, gives the Trigger Points room to relax, and for your client's ultimate relaxation.

We would like to believe that massage is the solution to relieving all pain but it is not. You will learn some natural pain relievers that are safe remedies for pain and inflammation that may also provide missing nutrients to help the body rebuild and repair itself.

Natural Anti-Inflammatories

Tips for Integrating Trigger Point Therapy into Your Massage Practice

This illustrated manual, Trigger Point Made Easy is yours to keep and make notes in.

2 ABOUT TRIGGER POINT THERAPY

All Trigger Point Therapy is based on the work by Dr. Janet Travell. Since then it has evolved. As you start taking classes on Trigger Point Therapy you will find that they all follow the same basic guidelines but they will all vary a little. A chiropractor teaching Trigger Point Therapy will have a different insight than a physical therapist versus a massage therapist or even an owner of a massage school. My guide to Trigger Point Therapy has been Bonnie Prudden's book, Pain Erasure. I have enhanced my knowledge by taking Trigger Point classes from massage schools and from The Institute of Trigger Point Therapy whose founder is a chiropractor.

WHAT IS A TRIGGER POINT?

A Trigger Point is a tender spot in the muscle (contracted muscle fiber).

1. It may have been caused from past injury.
2. Brought on by physical or emotional stress.
3. Maybe it is part of the muscular armor we develop as children to protect our self from social pressures or other suffering or abuse.
4. The birthing process. Your birth or you giving birth.
5. Recent injury.
6. Every day use of the body.
7. Develop from constantly working in awkward positions
8. Bad posture.
9. Muscle memory trying to protect itself from more injury
10. Being put in a awkward position during surgery, dental procedures, or medical tests
11. Part of the fight or flight response.

You are familiar with the fight or flight expression. Our bodies are designed to respond to any kind of danger whether it is a real physical danger or emotional stress. It sets off alarms to our nerves and hormones that prompt the adrenal glands to release hormones, such as adrenaline and cortisol.

This gives us extra energy by increasing the heart rate and blood pressure. Our bodies tense up. It tells our bodies to be ready to fight or run. Our breathing becomes concentrated in the top part of our chest. Since most of us are not out in the jungle facing a roaring lion and not on the battleground doing hand to hand combat, we have all this pent up energy with no way to release it.

A good way to release energy and adrenalin would be strenuous exercise, like running from a lion.

Deep breathing, breathing down in the belly area or diaphragm would signal our brain to tell the body to relax.

But we don't do either. Most of our stress is emotional or mental. Most of my clients come to me because they hurt, and it is not because they do hard physical work. It is stress. Rarely do I see clients that do hard physical work with Trigger Points. If they hurt it is because they have over worked or injured their muscles.

Muscles do 2 things. They either relax or they contract (tense up). That is how muscles move your body around. Contraction (tension) requires energy. If you stay tensed up all the time your muscles not only hurt from this constant tension but it drains your energy. Muscle tension requires energy just as though you were working. No wonder you are so tired.

Can you visualize your joints? Think of the elbow, you have the upper arm and the lower arm with the elbow in between. If the muscles in the upper arm and the lower arm are tensed and tight, they are both drawing at the elbow putting intense pressure on the elbow. That pressure on the joint is putting stress on the joints and the cartilage. Your body responds by creating inflammation. Guess what? Your elbow hurts. Same goes for the knees, hips and other joints. Is that arthritis?

If you have been under stress 24/7 your muscles (muscles have memory) have just forgotten how to relax. Your fight or flight response is not working properly.

These things create micro muscle spasms (muscle contractions), which may in turn lead to further micro muscle spasms and contractions. When muscles tighten in one spot it will pull on other muscles and can even pull vertebrae out of alignment. The results are chronic tension and pain.

You will always find another Trigger Point on the opposite side of the body. After working on the right side of your back or neck you will need to work on the left side of your back or neck.

Stand up. Lean to the right.

Notice the right side of your body is contracting while the left side of your body is stretching. If you hold the stretch long enough you may feel pain or tension on the left side of your body.

Where do you hurt?

Why do you hurt? Where does the pain start?

WHAT DOES A TRIGGER POINT FEEL LIKE?

When you apply pressure to a Trigger Point, you may feel a burning sensation or a sharp pain.
You may feel as if the area is bruised.
It may feel like a combination of all of the above.
Many times you will feel the pain radiate to distant areas.
The pain may be nauseating.
When searching for Trigger Points you are looking for a knot or a hard area in the muscle or a thickening in the muscle. The pain will let you know it when you find it.

HOW TO APPLY TRIGGER POINT PRESSURE?

Intense pressure is placed on the Trigger Point. The Bonnie Prudden's Way is for about 7-10 seconds. Other teachers will tell you 10-15 seconds. Others will say 5-7 seconds. And this will vary on different parts of the body.
The pressure is repeated 3-7 times.

This pressure is steady, gradually deepening as the spasm begins to let go and accepts more pressure.

You are not rubbing it in or rubbing around.

As you move around the Trigger Point you will find the most sensitive part of it.

Sometimes you can concentrate all your pressure on this area.

Sometimes it is so sensitive you have to work on the outside of it and work your way to the center. You need to breathe when you are doing this bodywork.
Sometimes you need to use less pressure and stay on the area longer.

When dealing with my pain, I stayed on each area for a full minute.

When you get through applying pressure, these knots will still be there. Doing this over and over will not make the knots go away. The area can be treated 3-5 times. The knots will still be there but you should feel like a little pressure or tension has let up or that the area is less tender. You will feel better the next day, and even better the day after that.

Many times I may treat the area 2-3 times, go to a different part of the body and then come back to it.

HOW MUCH PRESSURE?

You are using about 15-20 pounds of pressure on the neck and shoulder area, and 30-40 pounds on the gluteus or buttock area.

If you put a folded towel on the bathroom scale and press down you can determine the difference between 30-40 pounds and 15-20 pounds of pressure.
When applying pressure, you start lightly, gradually applying more and more pressure.
You apply as much pressure as you can take comfortably.

The idea is not how much pain you can endure but the most you can take comfortably. Your body should say, "oh that hurts so good." This should be on a pain scale of about a 7. Sometimes the area may be so sensitive that you can barely touch it.

You should breathe and relax into the pressure. If you are holding your breath, that is too much pressure.

DO NOT APPLY TRIGGER POINT THERAPY TO:

Inflamed or swollen areas
Recently injured
Bruised areas

You can apply Trigger Point therapy around and leading up to an injury. When you injure yourself, other muscles jump in to keep you from using that muscle. Releasing the Trigger Point in these other muscles will help relax the muscles and reduce the pain.

WHY DOES TRIGGER POINT WORK?

There are many theories why Trigger Point works. Dr. Janet Travell, the originator of Trigger Point, says it works because you are cutting off the oxygen supply to the Trigger Point, causing the muscle to relax due to an inability to continue to work.

For example, when our leg is deprived of good circulation a tingling sensation occurs: we often say "my leg fell asleep." The tingling is the return of oxygen. However you may have noticed the leg is difficult to use until ample oxygen has returned to the area. It may be that the Trigger Point method is utilizing this same concept in a smaller area. You are using firm steady pressure to cut off circulation to the Trigger Point. If you are rubbing it, you are defeating your purpose by increasing circulation.

Others have compared Trigger Point to acupressure, in which enough pressure is applied to block the transmission of impulses from the brain to the muscle, forcing the muscle to relax.

Richard Hoff has a different explanation. He says, "Muscle spasms are contractions of the muscle fibers. Muscle fibers contract, or shorten, by thickening. This is how muscles move your body around. If you then apply a steady, compressing pressure against the thickened muscle fibers, it is harder for them to maintain the contraction, and they are induced to let go and relax. This is also why stretching helps muscles to relax. When you stretch a muscle you are contradicting the contraction by lengthening it. Pressure, then, contradicts this contraction from the other direction, by pressing down against the thickening. Stretching and pressure point massage are natural allies in the alleviation of muscle tension."

Stretching, taking a hot bath or a heating pad prior to doing Trigger Point Therapy will help reduce soreness from the therapy.
You definitely will want to take a hot bath afterwards and drink plenty of water.

Beginning your massage with effleurage or gliding strokes prior to Trigger Point Therapy accomplishes this same purpose. The long gliding strokes warms up the skin and muscles while stretching the fascia and muscles. This helps the client to relax and helps you locate problem areas. You also finish with effleurage or gliding strokes to clear and soothe the treated area.

3 THE THERA CANE FOR THE UPPER BODY

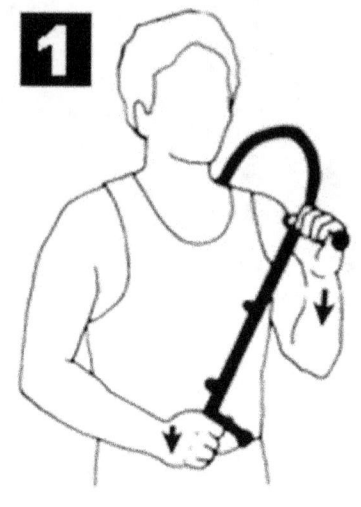

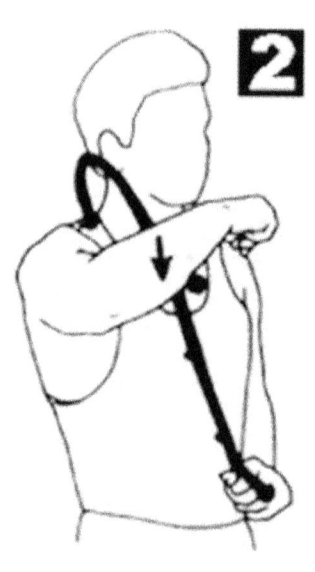

Hook over right shoulder, placing the ball on top of the shoulder.

Right hand on top handle.

Left hand on end of the Thera Cane

Pull down with left hand wiggling the Thera Cane around until you find a trigger point.

Using the left hand, pull straight down, then, pull up. Notice the pressure will become deeper.
Keeping the pressure up, try sliding the Thera Cane around the skin to different parts of the muscles.

Always use the opposite hand for the pressure. The other hand is for balance.

Switch hands and try the same thing. Notice you are putting stress on the shoulder you are trying to relax.

Raise your right arm and relax it on the top handle of the Thera Cane.

Change sides and feel the difference.

There are other ways to use the Thera Cane. This is just to get you started.

You can also sit in a chair and lean into the Thera Cane.

THIS IS A GUIDE

Each body is unique, with its own pain patterns and causes. It is not important to know exact locations of Trigger Points, but to know the general area to search for the Trigger Points.

Once you learn how to do Trigger Point, use your imagination to perfect your own techniques.

Muscles are paired, always work the paired muscle on the opposite side of the body.

Start with 7-10 seconds of pressure. As you get to know your body you can increase the pressure and length of time. You may eventually need to spend a full minute on a stubborn location. One client told me that if she can press a Trigger Point site located in her shoulder long enough, she can stop a migraine headache.

If a Trigger Point is really sensitive, using less pressure for a longer period of time can be more effective.

If you are using so much pressure that your body tenses up you are being counter- productive. You must be able to relax into the pressure. Breathe.

Changing body positions such as rotating the neck or bending the neck to the right or to the left will allow you access to different muscles and allow attacking the Trigger Point at different angles.

Changing arm positions while working on the shoulder blade area or bending the leg while working on the hip area can be crucial to success.

Your muscles are in layers. Your pain is in layers. As you begin your work you will be releasing satellite pain and referred pain. As you continue to work these areas you will gradually release deeper layers of knots until your pain centralizes. Once your pain centralizes, you can focus on the source of the pain, your main Trigger Point.

After a Trigger Point session, stretch the treated area.
A stretch must be held for 6 seconds to be effective.

Drink water and take a hot bath.
Your muscles may be sore. If you hurt, you have toxins. When you do this bodywork you are releasing toxins into your system. It is very important to drink a lot of water to flush the toxins out of your system and to take a hot bath that night. The bath will be more effective if you add either 1 cup of Epsom Salts or ½ cup of apple cider vinegar to the bath.

You will not feel relief the first day.
You will not receive 100% relief the first day. The nerves are irritated and will take a day to heal. When you pull a piece of glass out of your foot, your foot still hurts even though the glass has been removed. The nerves are irritated. Trigger Points are like that piece of glass. Your body may still hurt even though you have released the Trigger Points.

Do Not be Overwhelmed by the many Trigger Points Illustrated.

The first day may take an hour just to locate your individual Trigger Points. Future treatments will take only minutes to work, once you know your individual Trigger Points. After the satellite Trigger Points have been released, you may have only one or two Trigger Points to deal with on a regular basis. Releasing these Trigger Points at the first sign of tension will prevent "flare ups". Trigger Points can change according to your activities.

Carolyn Gibson

TRIGGER POINT SITES FOR THE NECK, SHOULDERS AND HEADACHE CAUSED BY NECK TENSION

Trigger Points for these areas begin with the Trapezius.

Tension in this large diamond shape muscle can prevent you from reaching Trigger Points in underlying muscles. Remember your pain is in layers.

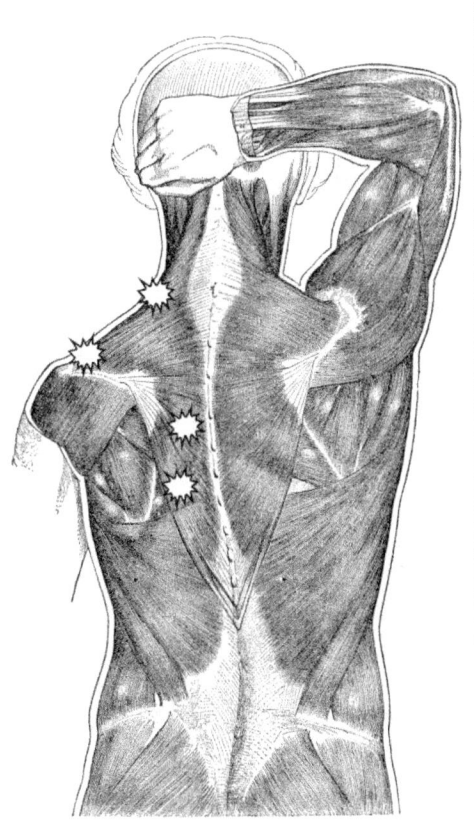

Trapezius
Trigger Points

Contributes to pain on the back and side of the neck,

Between the shoulder blades, And top of the shoulder.

Can be cause of tension and migraine headaches

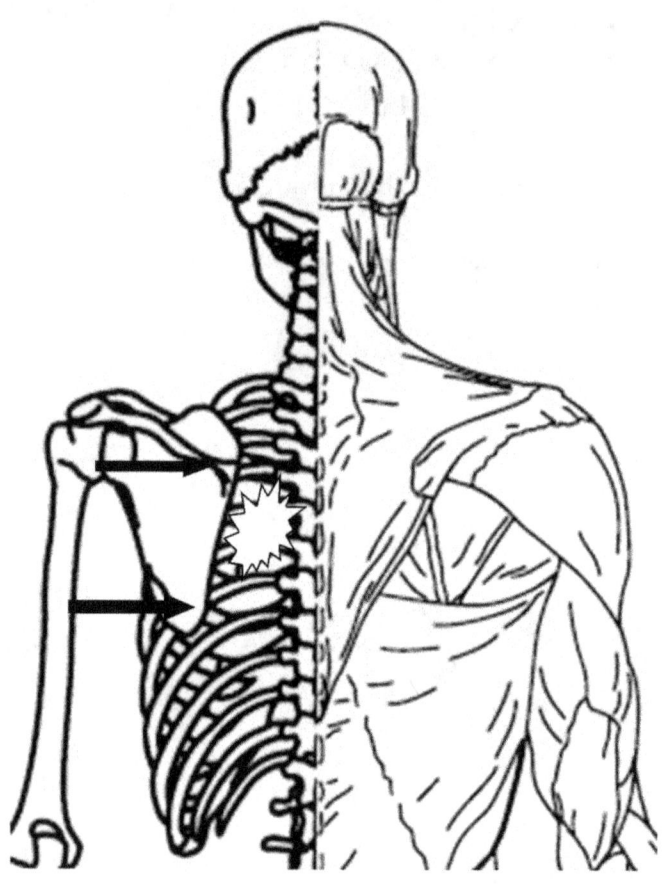

Lower Trapezius

This is the first spot we naturally head for.
Begin your Trigger Point Search by releasing the Lower
Trapezius, located halfway between the shoulder blade and
the spine. Notice the 2 arrows on the shoulder blade.

THERA CANE AND THE LOWER TRAPEZIUS

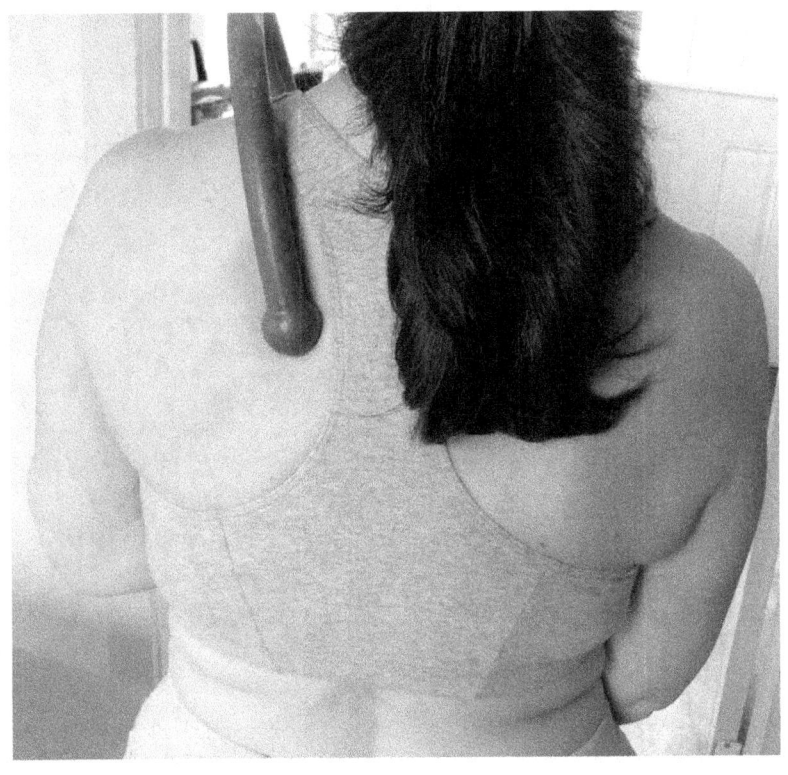

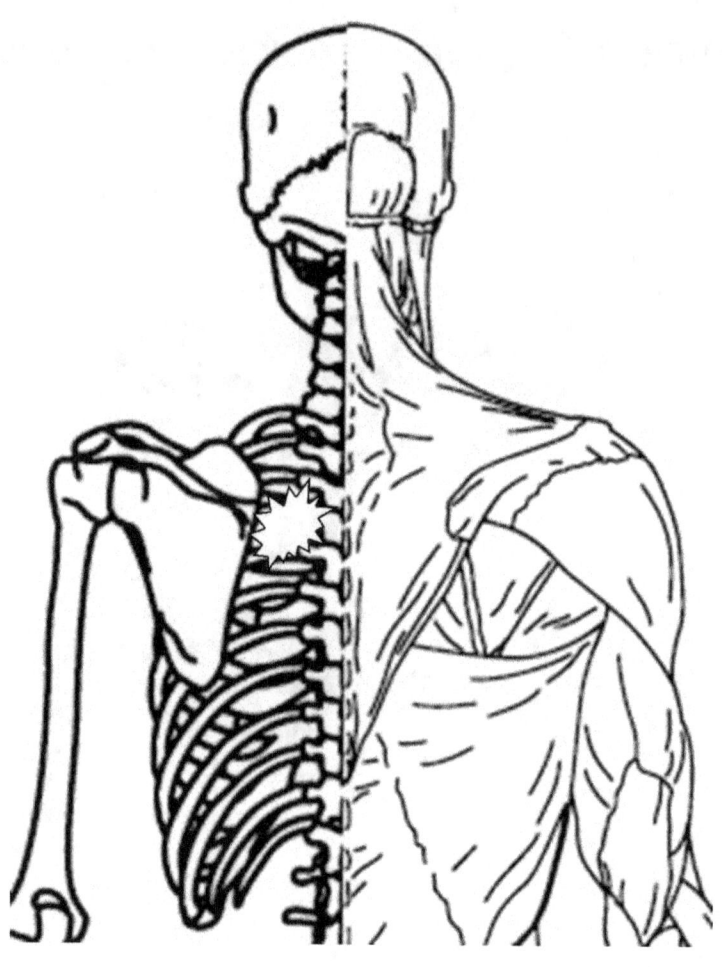

Middle Trapezius

Search for the Middle Trapezius Trigger Point right above the Lower Trapezius.

THERA CANE AND THE MIDDLE TRAPEZIUS

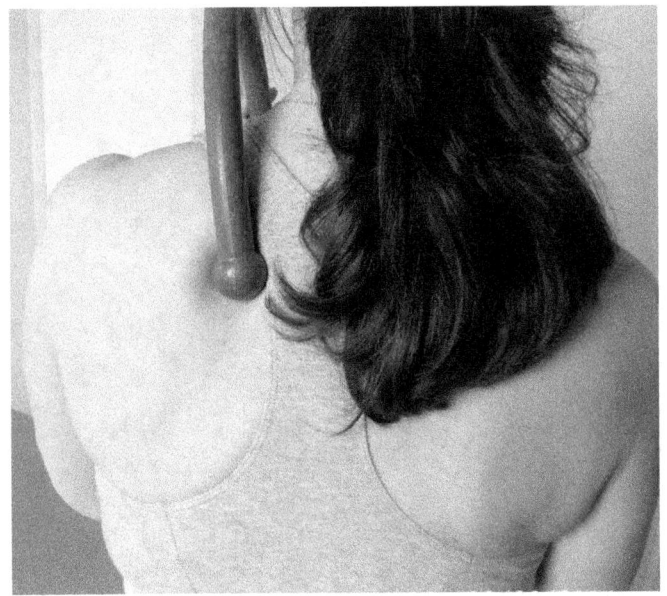

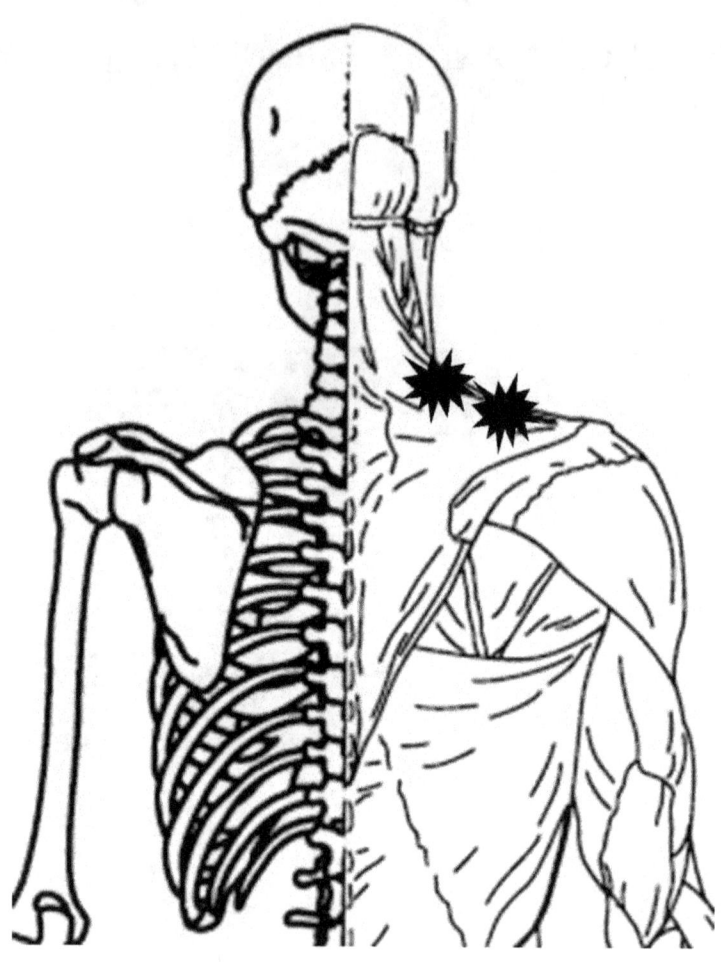

Upper Trapezius

Start next to the neck and work across. This is a really thick muscle.

THERA CANE AND THE UPPER TRAPEZIUS

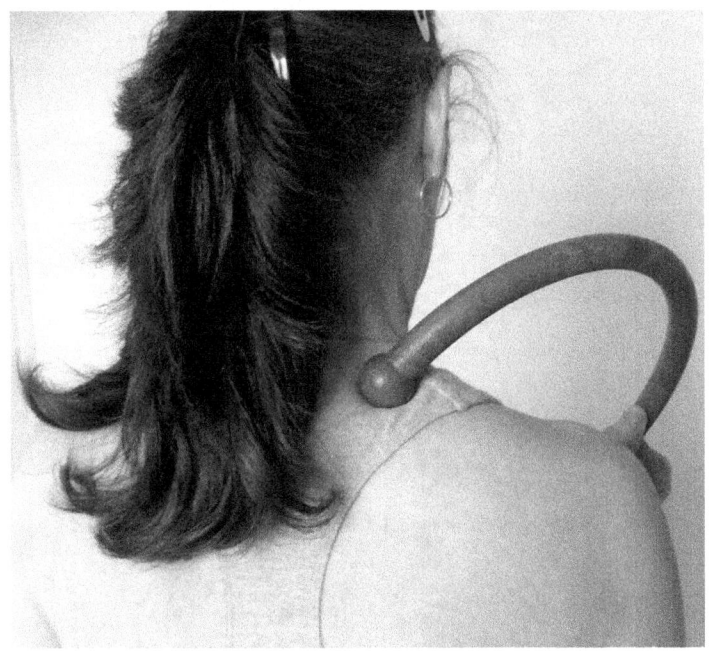

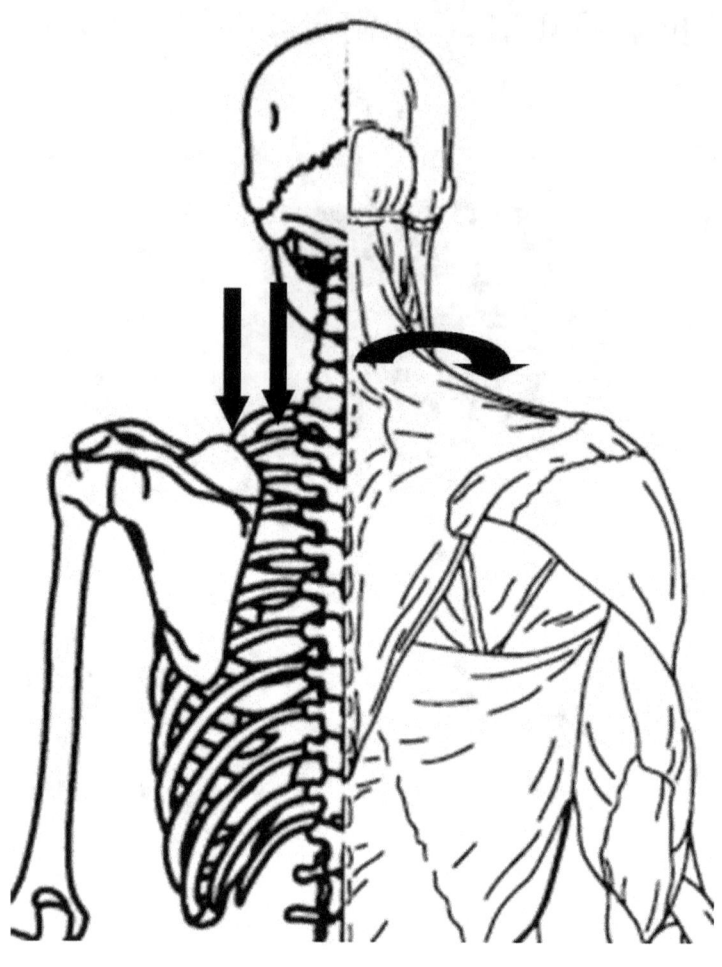

The Levator Scapulae Trigger Points lies under the Upper Trapezius along the groove of the shoulder and refers pain to the neck and upper back.

THERA CANE AND LEVATOR SCAPULAE

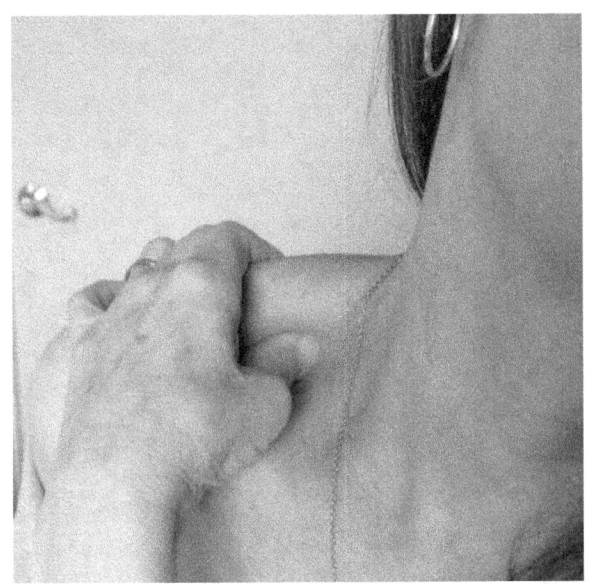

This can be difficult to reach with self treatment

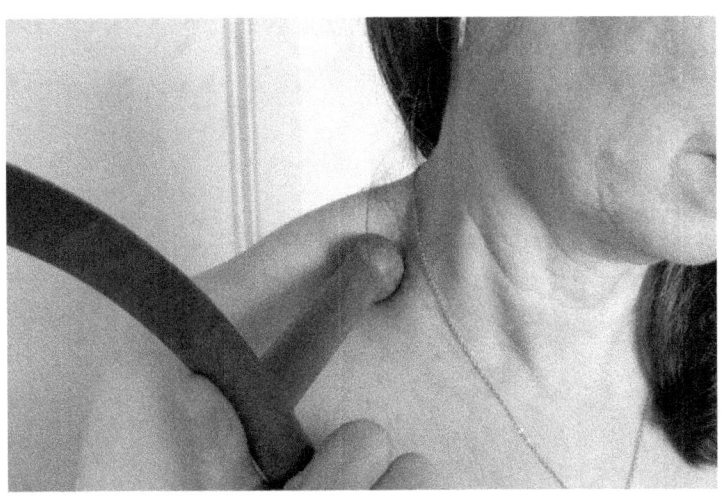

TOP SHOULDER BLADE SPINE

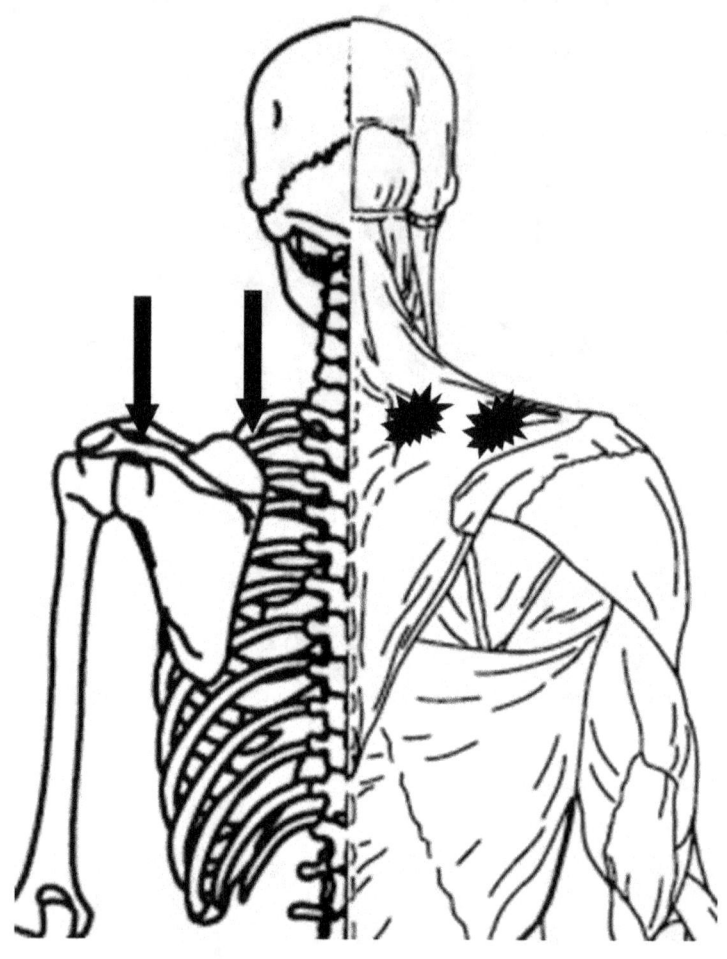

Search across the top spine of the shoulder blades

THERA CANE AND TOP OF THE SHOULDER BLADE

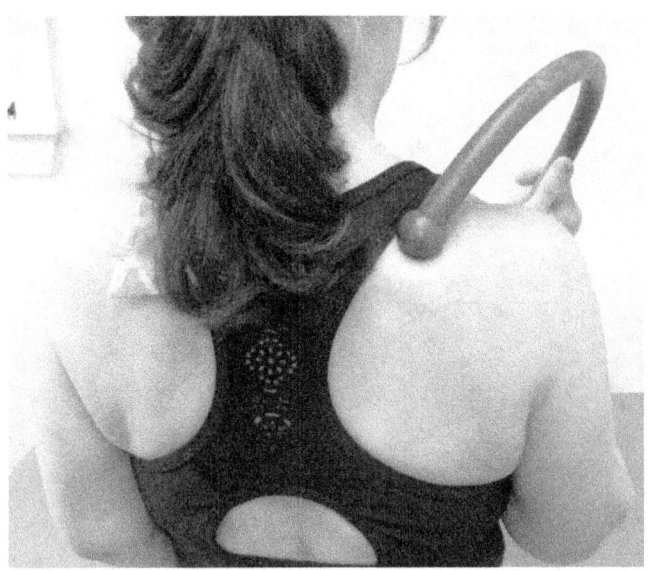

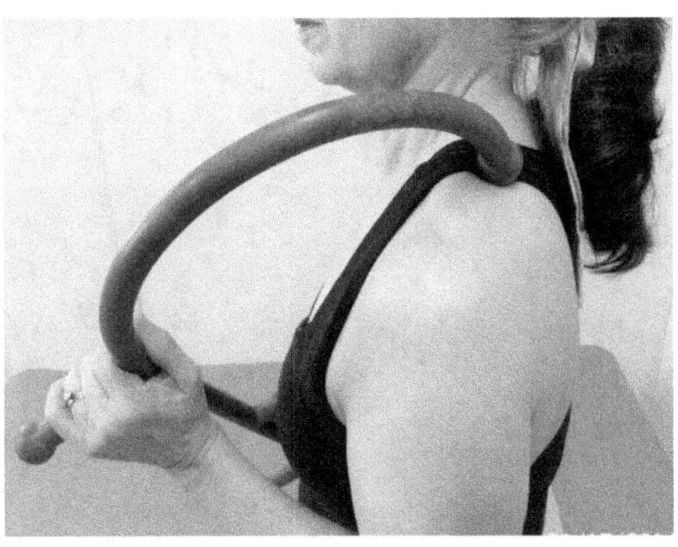

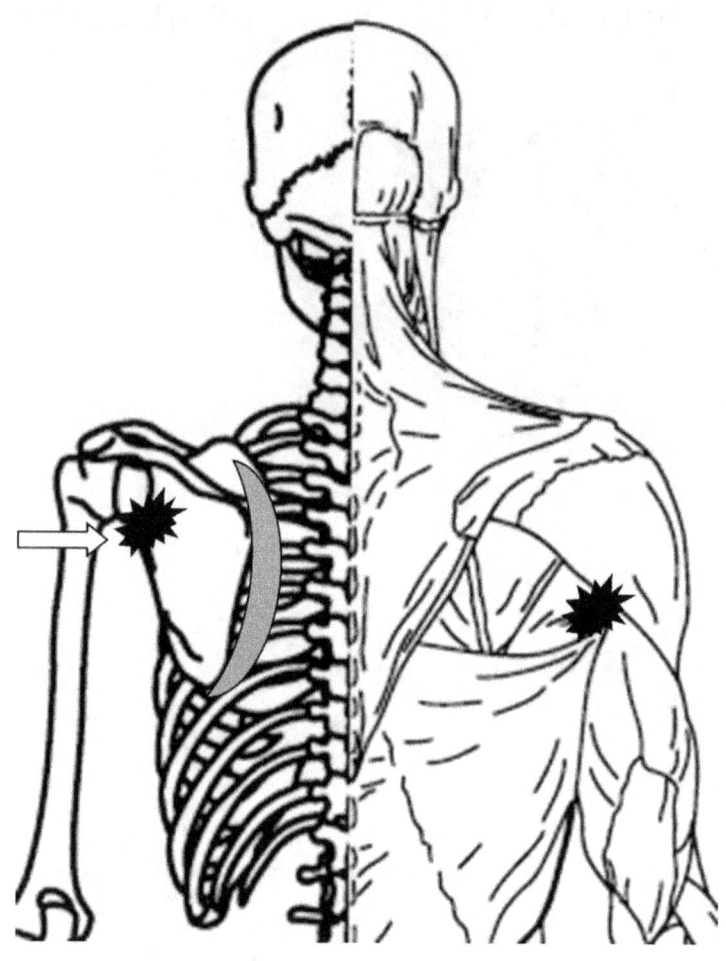

The Rhomboids lie under the Trapezius along the edge of the shoulder blade. See gray area.
Search all around the shoulder blade, underneath, on top, and above.
Notice the spot by the arm, often over looked as a cause of neck pain.

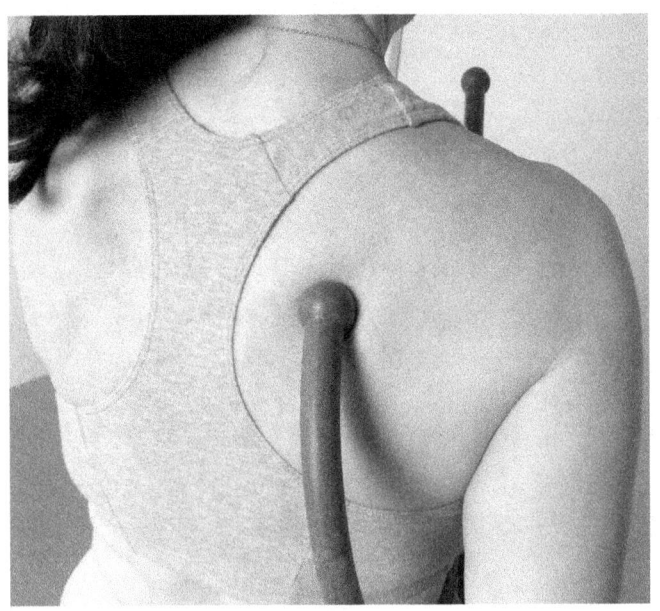

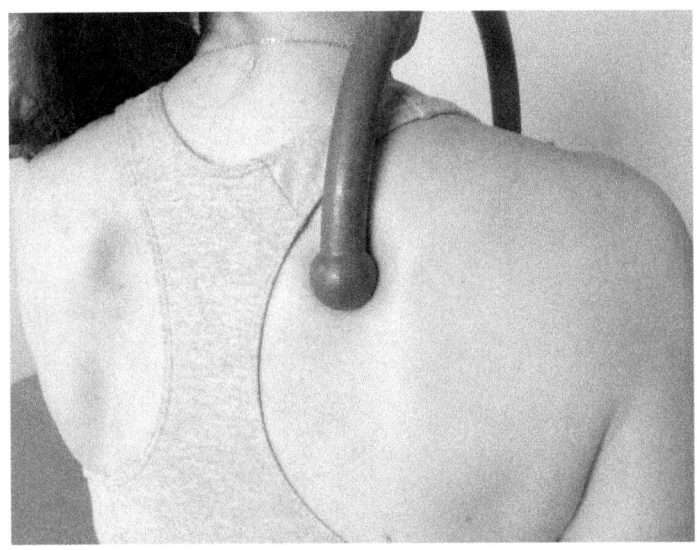

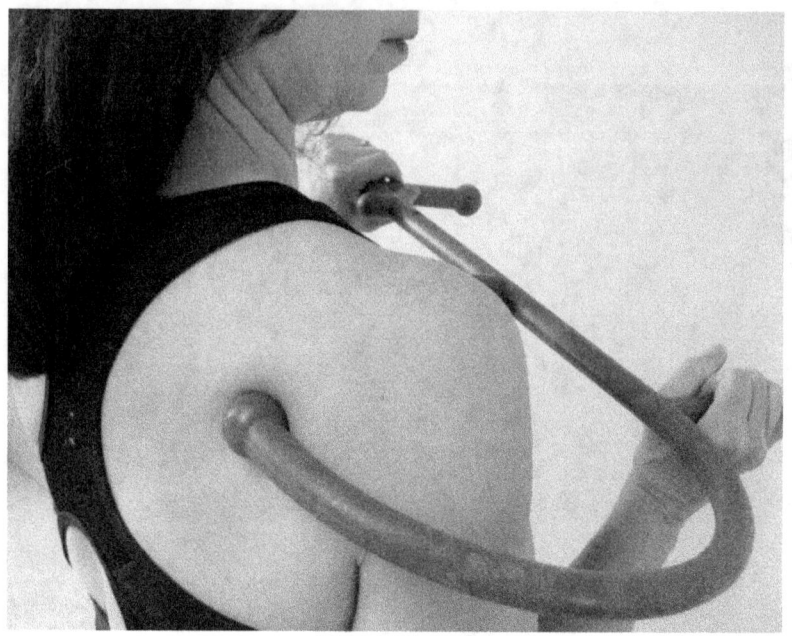

THE STERNOCLEIODMASTOID

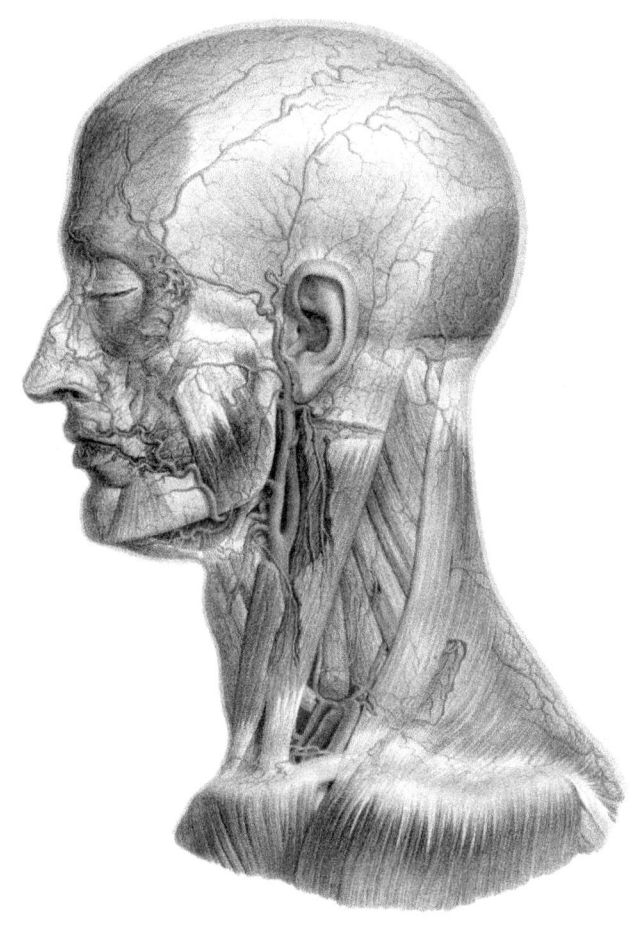

STERNOCLEIDOMASTOID

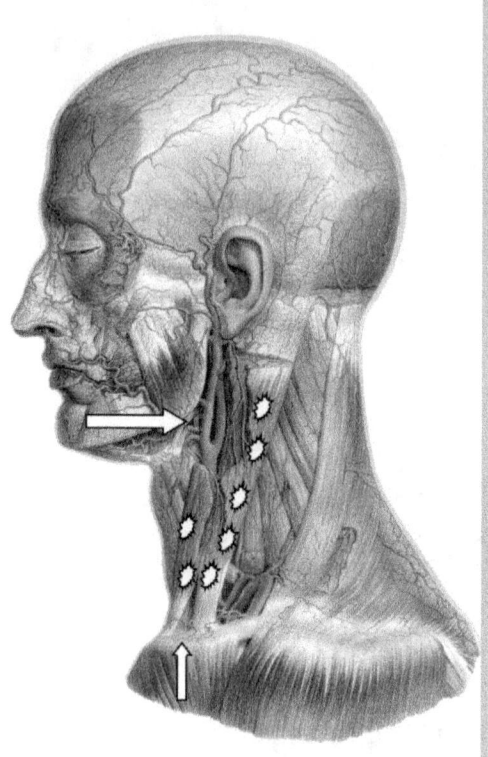

This may be the cause of cluster, vascular and migraine headaches.

Pain may be felt around the eye sockets,

On top, and the back of the head and the forehead.

May cause dizziness, nausea, scratchy throat and dry cough,

Vision problems,

Sea or car sickness

Fingers are used to knead this area. When you find an area of tension hold for 3-5 seconds. Go up and down 3-4 times.

Notice there are 2 parts to this muscle, the Sternal division and the Clavicular division.

Caution: There are many blood vessels and nerves trunks running through this area. Remember light pressure.

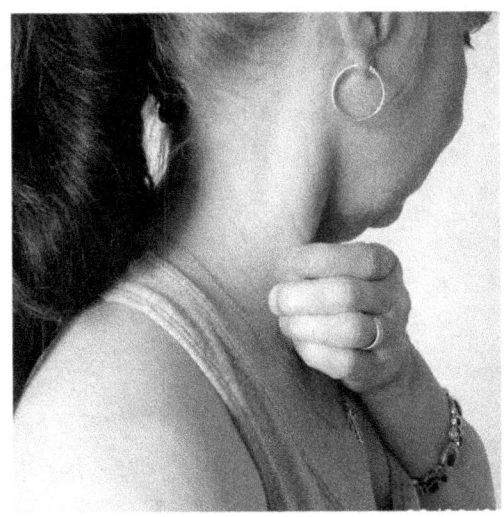

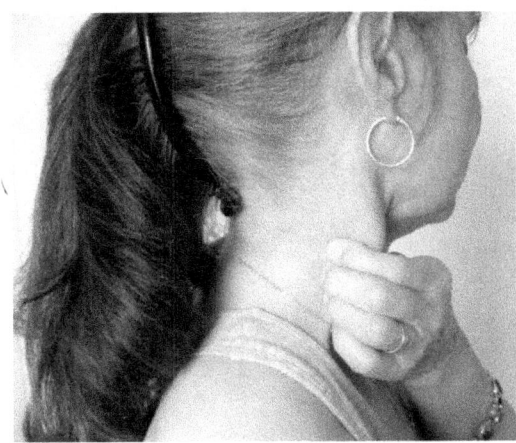

Turn your neck and feel for this muscle. You can easily find the Sterno division, it is a little harder to find the Clavicular division. When working on your clients this muscle is easier to locate in the side position.

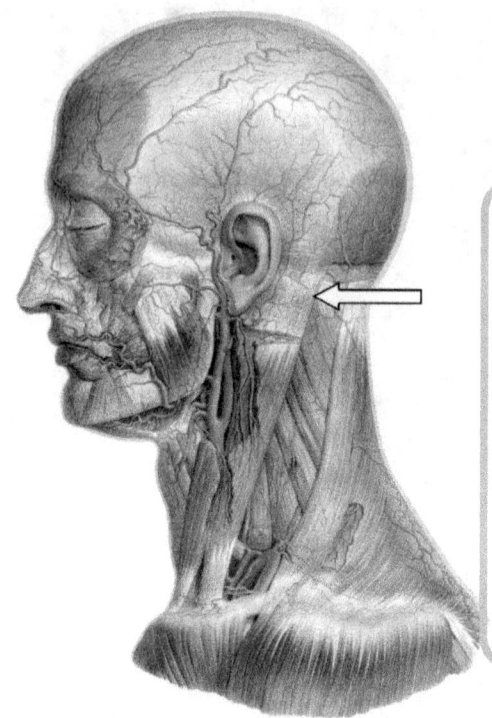

Right behind the Sternocleidmastoid, under the Mastoid Process about 1-2 inches lie a Trigger Point that will require deep pressure.

You can use the Thera Cane or the Knobble. Your pressure is directed towards the nose, not up towards the head.

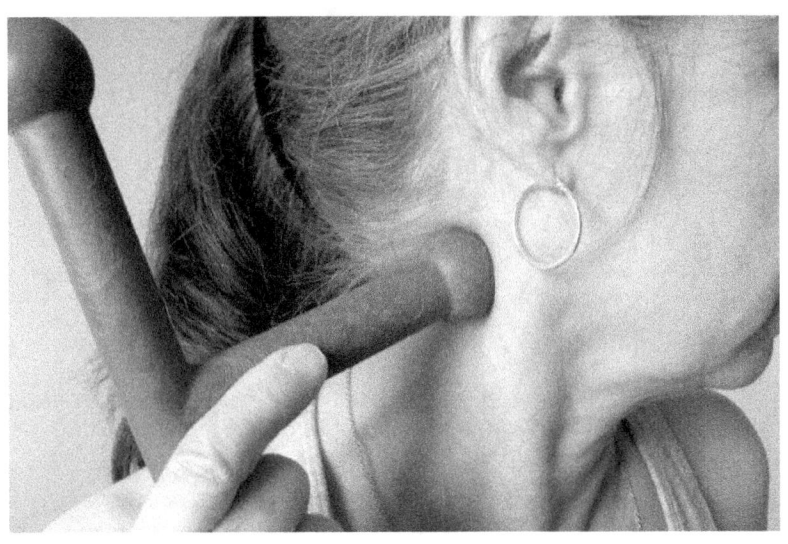

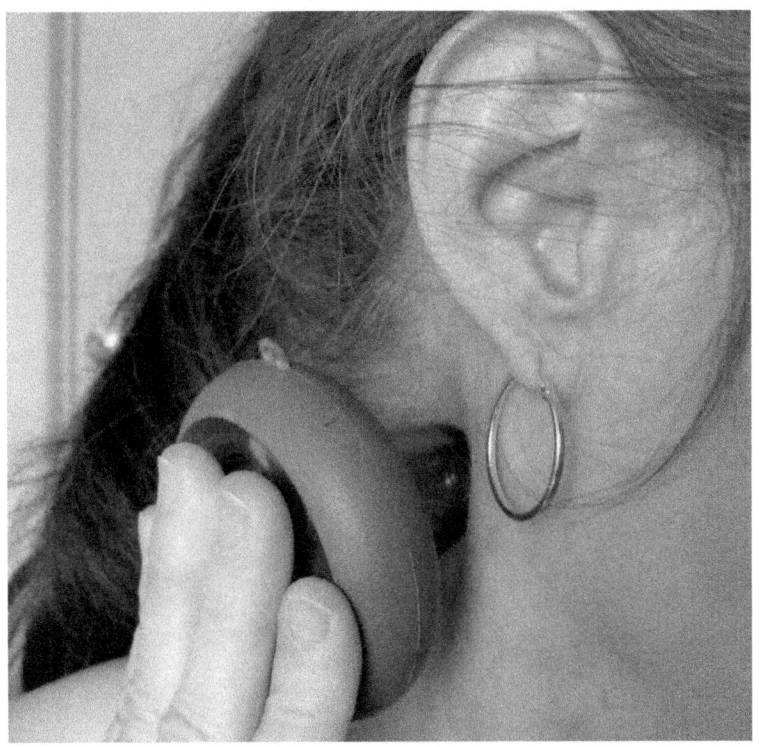

OTHER NECK AREAS

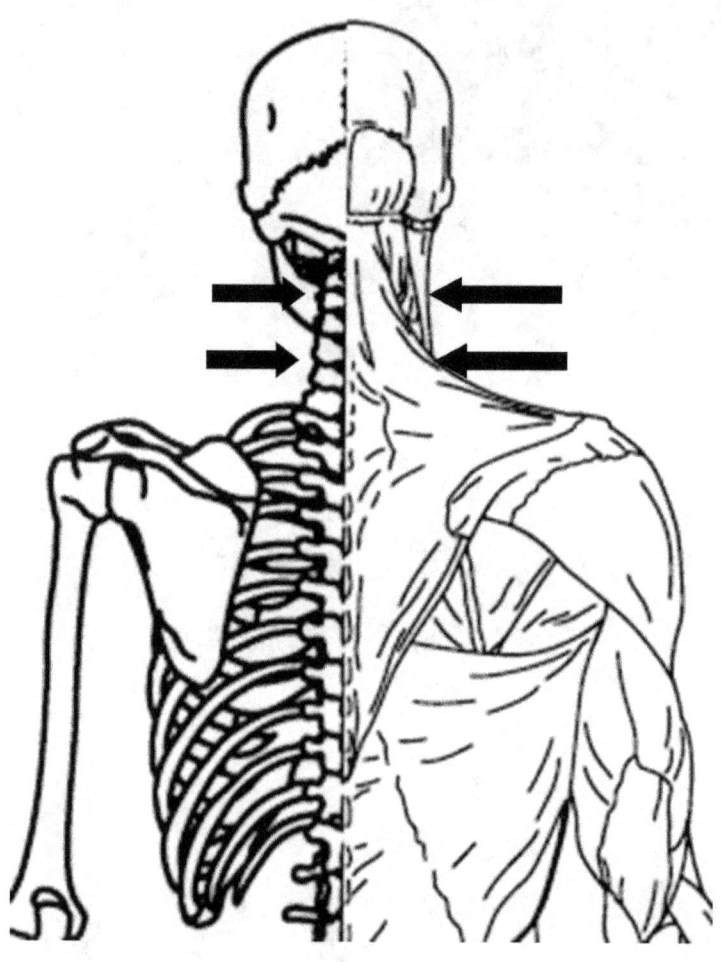

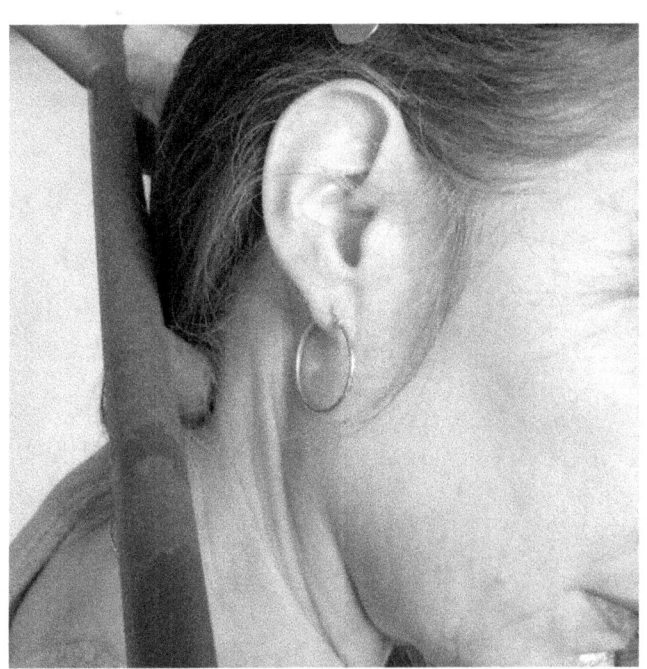

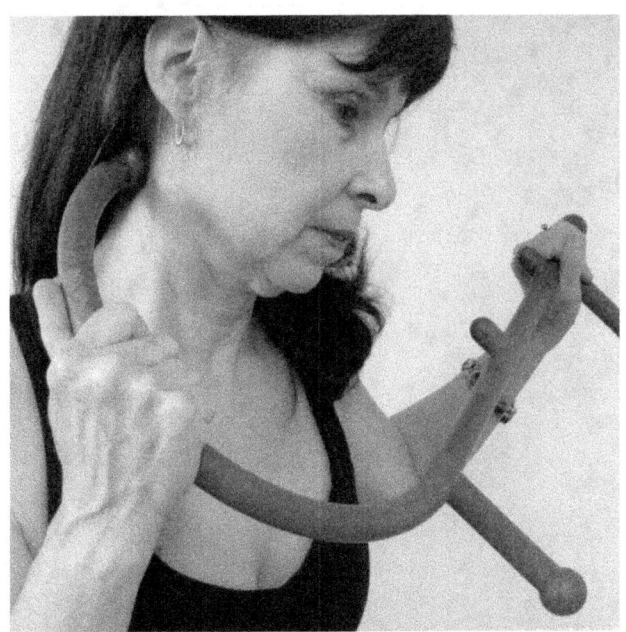

BACK AND SIDE OF SKULL

Does anyone remember how many muscles there are in the skull?
Do you think the skull has Trigger Points?

Yes they have many Trigger Points. We will cover a few of them.

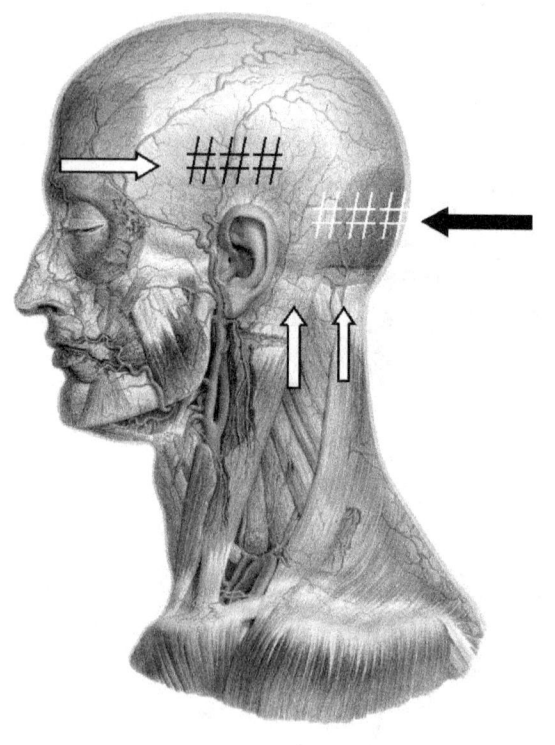

Go upward under the curve of the skull from ear to ear. You will find spots that are nauseating and may radiate to other areas. Search for Trigger Points behind the skull and on the side of the skull.

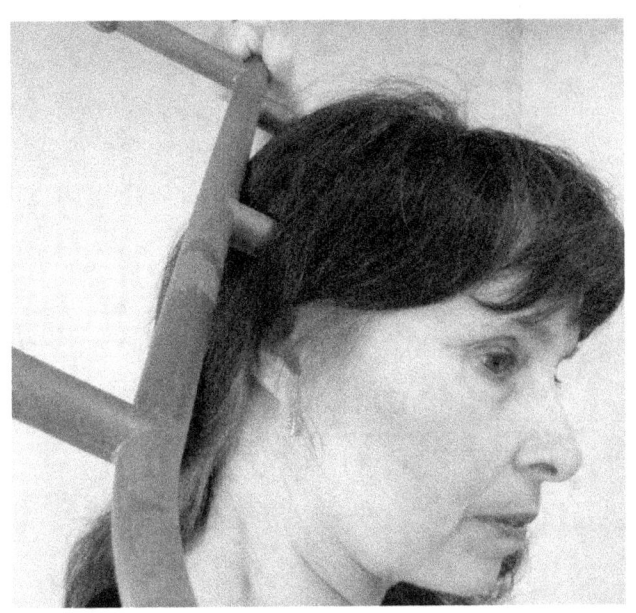

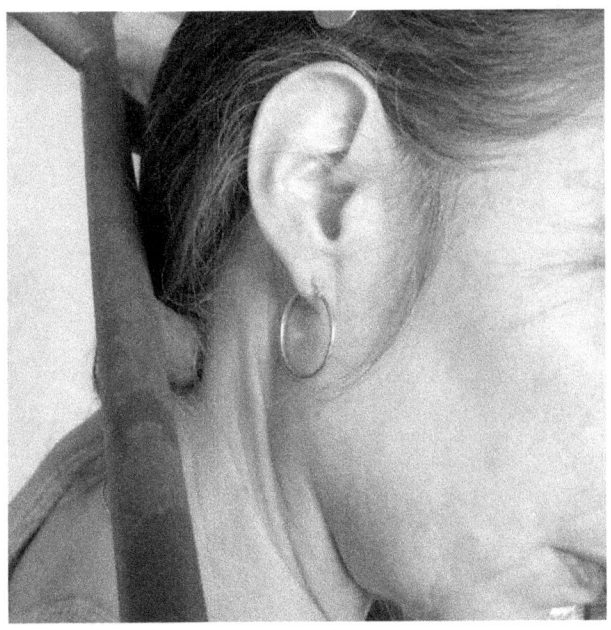

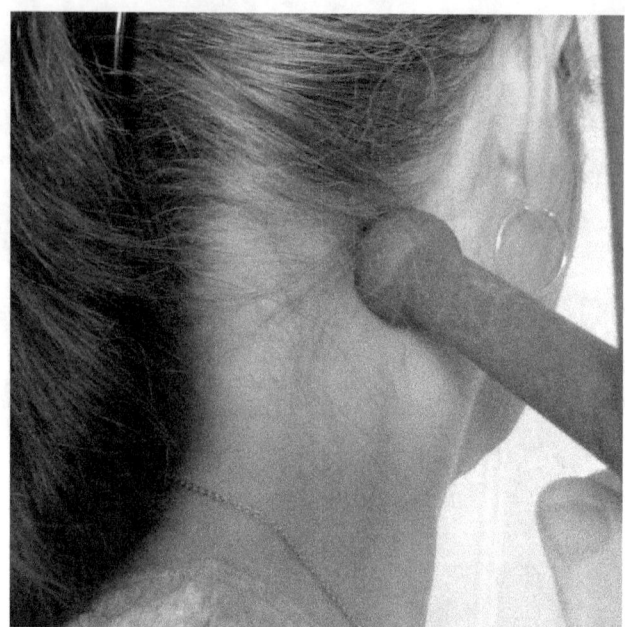

Apply pressure upwards when under the curve of the skull.

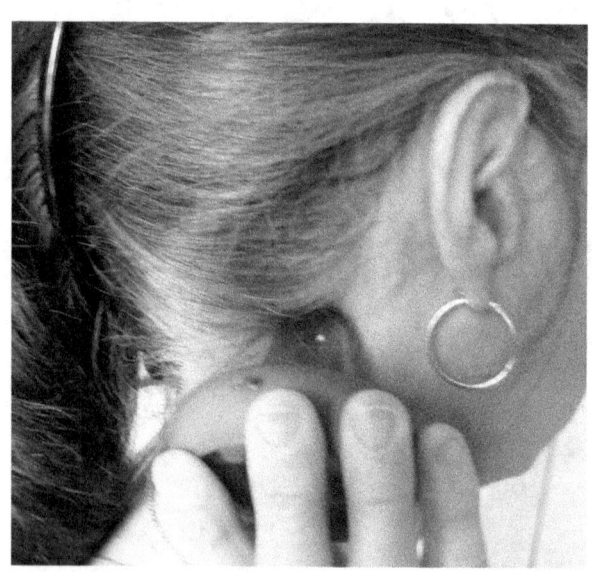

4 SCIATICA, LOW BACK, HIPS AND HIP JOINTS AND PAIN DOWN THE LEG

The Trigger Points illustrated located in the pelvis or buttock area will treat low back pain and sciatic nerve pain. The Trigger Points in the legs are also for Sciatic Nerve Pain.

SCIATICA: TOSSIN N TURNING

Sciatic nerve pain, this is the pain in the buttocks, or in your hip, or hip joint. It can go down either side of your leg or behind your leg. This is the pain that keeps you tossing and turning all night trying to get comfortable. This is the pain that can make a car ride or a plane trip torture. Forget sitting. You can either stand, walk, or lie down, but not for very long. You just keep alternating. You know what I mean if you have it.

It is brought on by prolonged sitting, bending over, or lifting heavy objects. It may be brought on by the slightest increase in shoe heel height, or worn out heels on your shoes.

Remember what I said about your pelvis being your center of balance.

Any circumstances causing you to tense up the muscles in your buttocks or leg muscles can cause sciatic nerve pain.

It could be unresolved emotional issues creating this tension.

Sciatic nerve pain can also be caused by compression of the lumbar disc.

In my experience it is a combination of both.

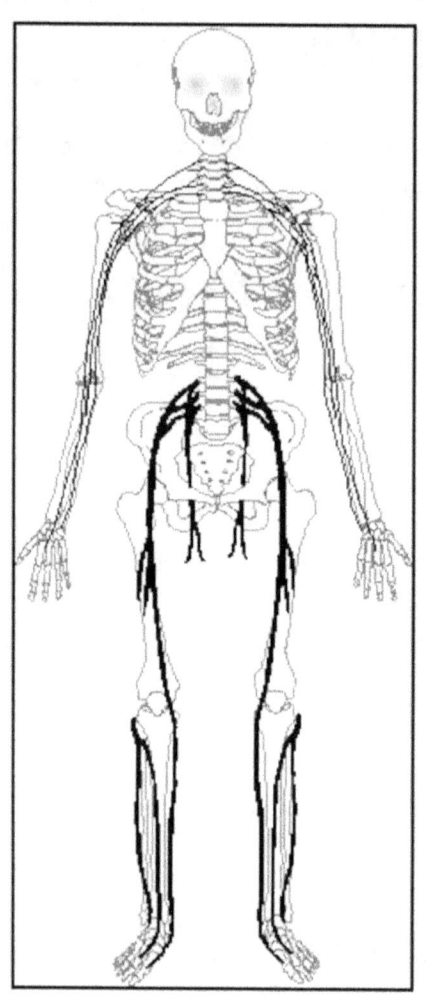

The sciatic nerve start at L-4, goes through the sacrum (the tailbone), continues through the muscles in the buttocks, Gluteus Maximus, Medius and Minimus and the Piriformis, and then runs along the hip joints, then goes on down through the thigh splitting at the knee and down to the feet.

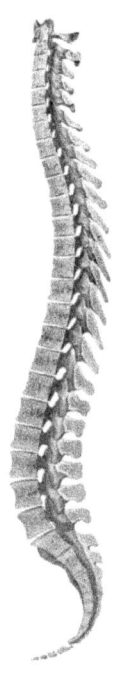

> The spinal column is made up of 24 vertebrae.
>
> There are 7 in the neck, the chest area has 12, and the low back is made up of 5 vertebrae, the tailbone being the largest.

The low back area is called the lumbar region. Correct posture maintains the curve in the lumbar region keeping the front angle of the vertebrae open and maintains balance of the low back muscles.

Bad posture and bending over closes this opening and over-stretches the low back muscles.

The results are a bulging or herniated disc causing compression of the sciatic nerve and overstretched muscles. If one set of muscles are overstretched than means the opposing muscles are being shortened or compressed (tensed).

If compression of the lumbar disc is causing your sciatic nerve pain, then Body Arching may relieve your pain if your condition has not progressed too far. Body Arching will come later in the book.

Carolyn Gibson

We will treat muscle tension caused by the Trigger Points in the buttock and leg area with the Knobble.

Don't let that point scare you.

You can use either the edge of the Knobble II or the point depending on how much pressure that you need.

The point also stabilizes the Knobble when it is turned on its side.

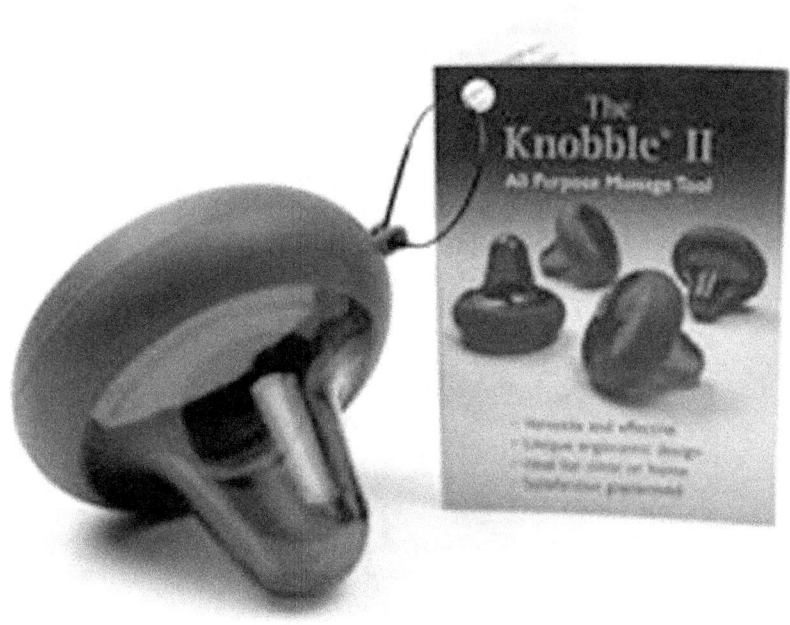

THE KNOBBLE FOR
TRIGGER POINTS FOR SCIATICA AND LOW BACK PAIN

The buttock area contributes both to lower back pain and sciatic pain. This area takes a lot of pressure. Even though the Thera Cane can be used I prefer the Knobble for this body work. Lying on the floor with the Knobble uses your own body weight for the pressure.

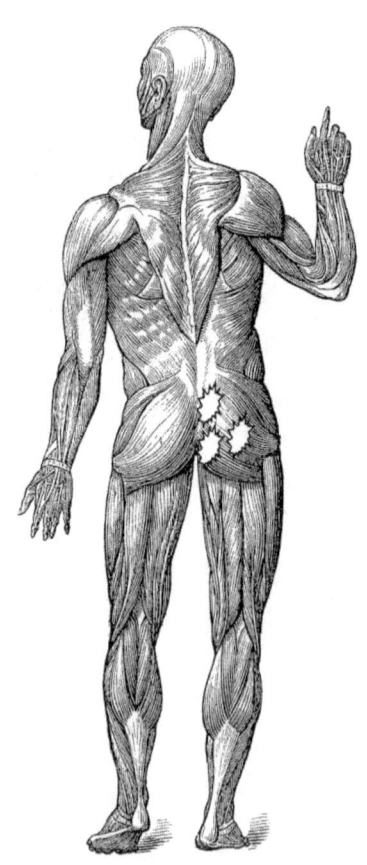

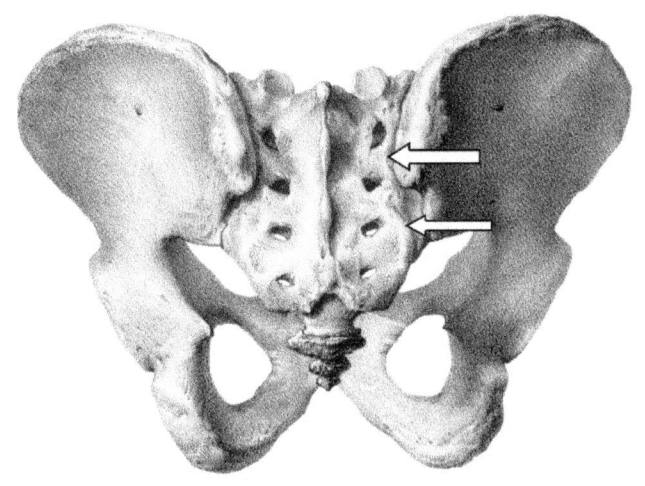

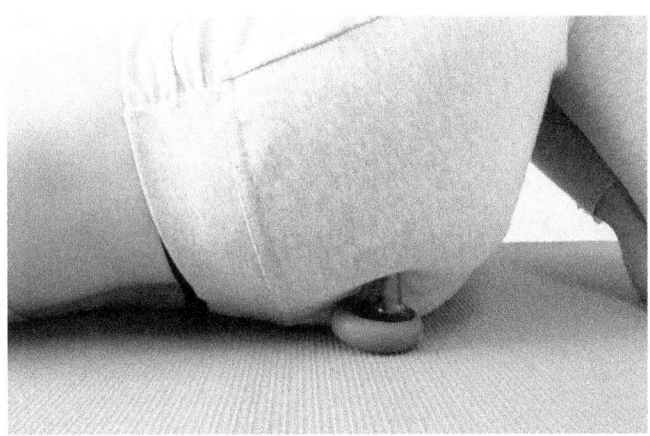

Search for Trigger Points on the edge of the sacrum, angling your pressure up against the sacrum.

Carolyn Gibson

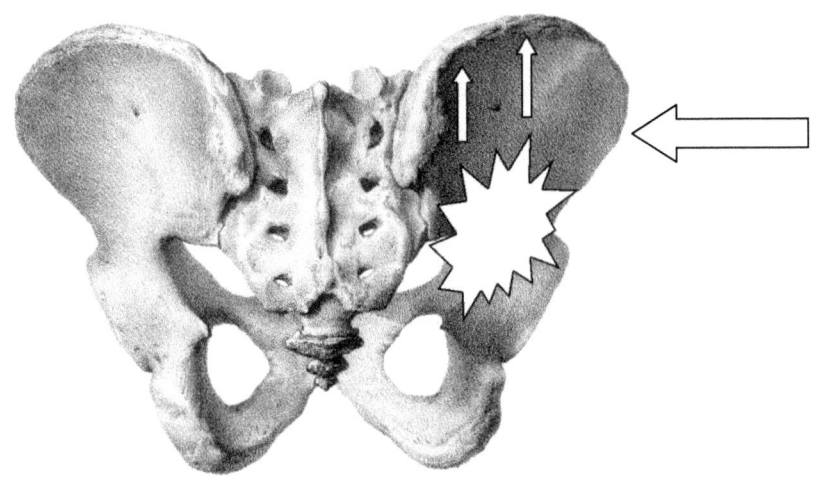

Trigger Points are where your back pocket would be. Search the whole area. Also search up into the iliac crest. Go to the edge of your buttocks. These may lie almost on the side of your buttocks.

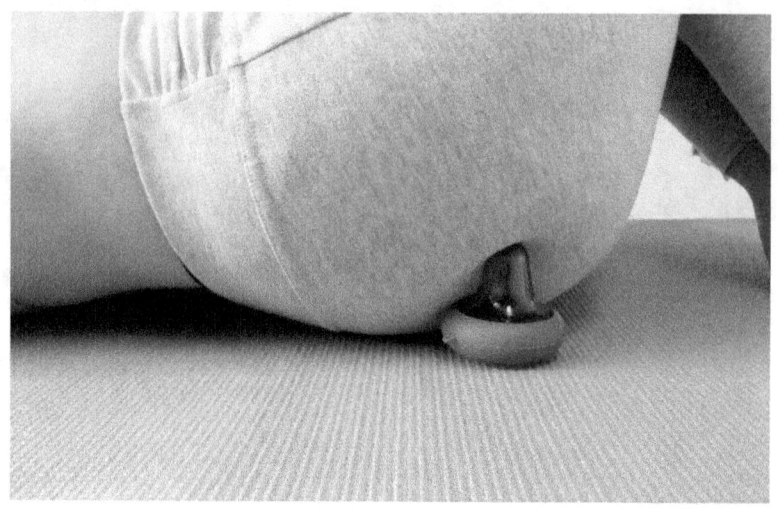

You may need to lean slightly over to your side.

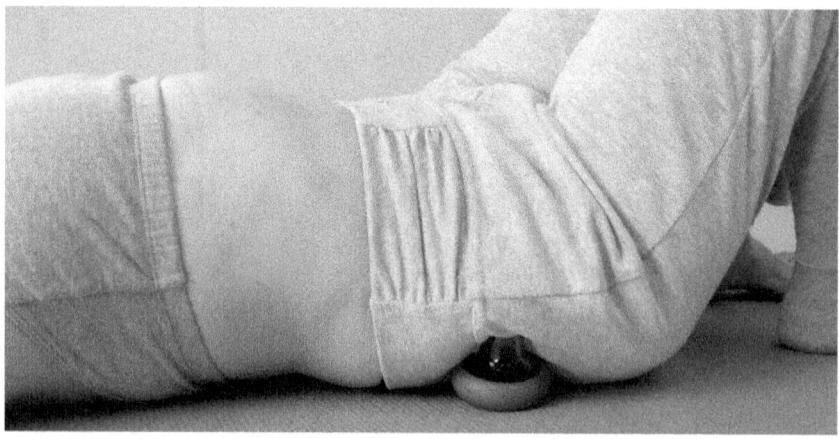

Different leg positions will help attack the muscles at different angles. You can bend the leg at the knee with your feet on the floor or try bending the leg and the knee and lowering the knee to the floor at a right angle. Or as I like to call it, the frog.

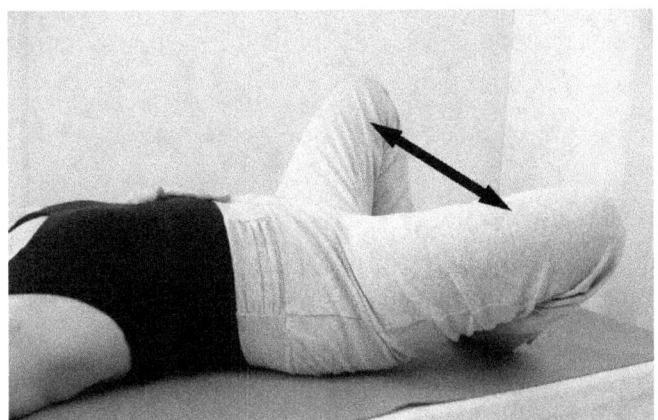

Search across the waist line. You will work next to the spine and go across in each direction but not on the spine. Beside the spine is really fine, but never, never, on top of the spine.

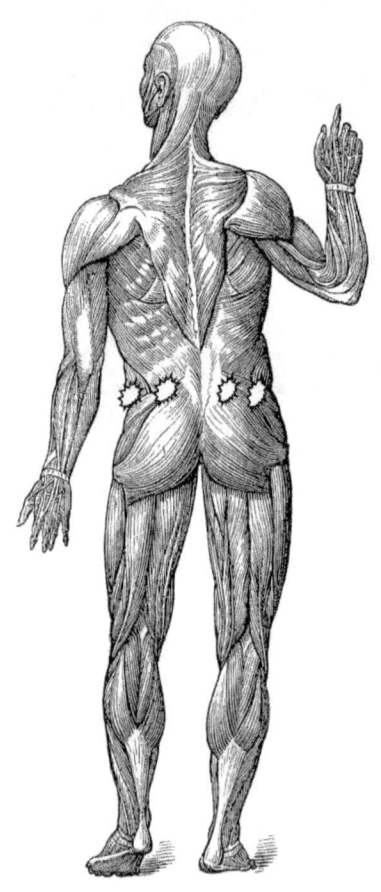

KNOBBLE GOING ACROSS THE WAIST

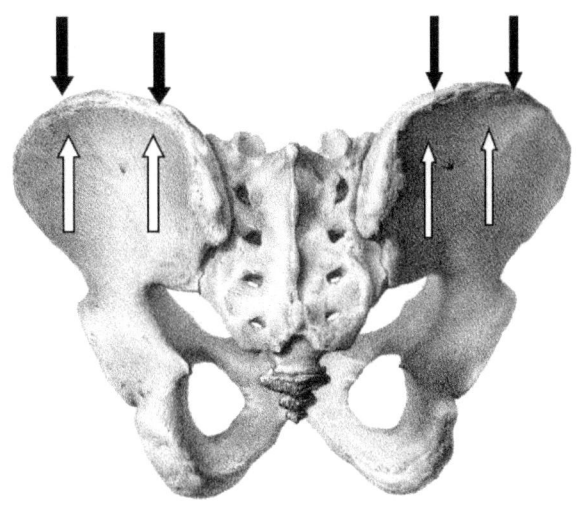

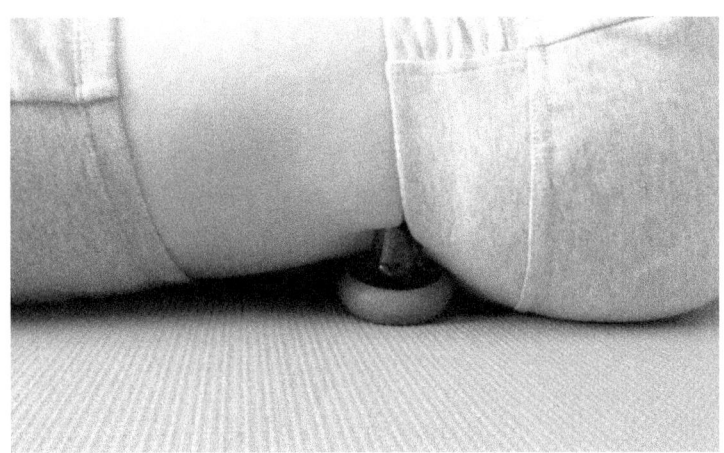

TRIGGER POINTS IN THE LEG FOR SCIATICA

The Thera Cane could be used for these but I prefer the Knobble II or for you that are really sensitive you can use a small ball or a tennis ball. The outside and inside of the leg has many Trigger Points. These Trigger Points can be the cause of hip pain and sciatica.

Imagine you are wearing a jogging suit with a runner stripe. There will be Trigger Points running along the "runner stripe" on the outside of the leg and the inside of the leg. Some of these can also be responsible for knee pain.

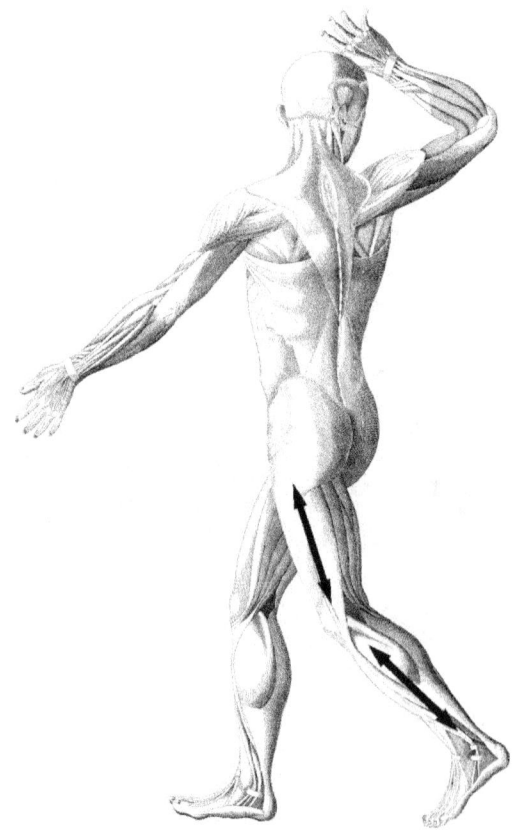

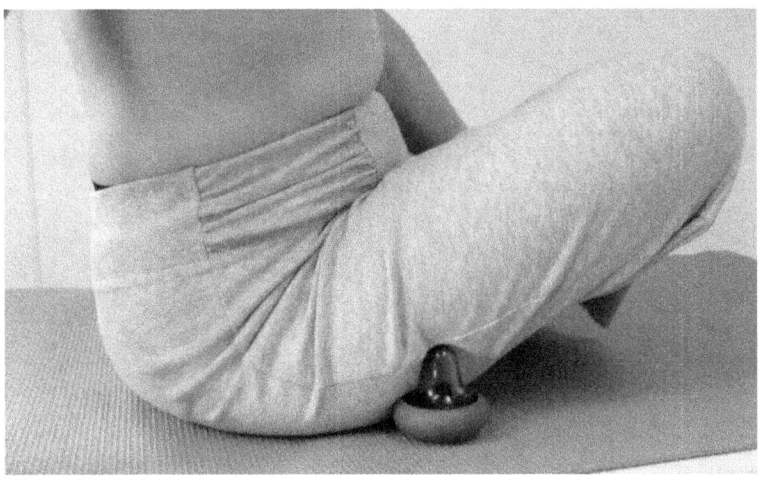

Simply sit on the floor and use your body weight against the Knobble II. When you start applying pressure you will know that you are in the right spot. Work your way down to the knee.

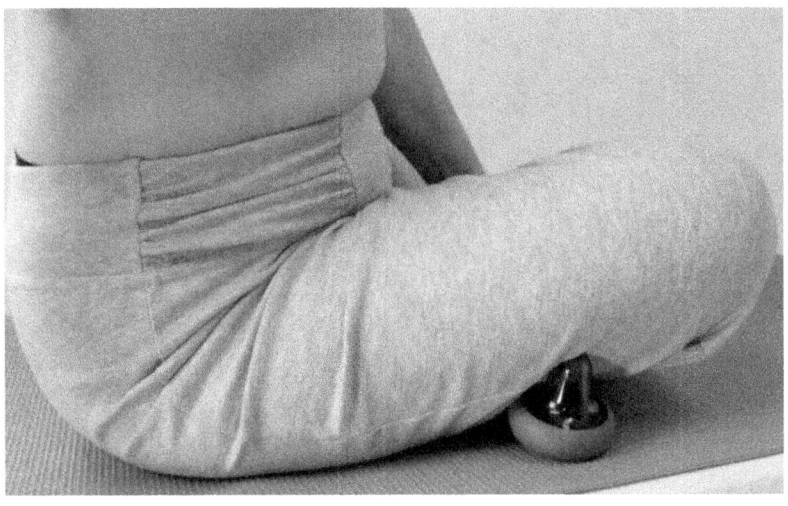

Carolyn Gibson

INSIDE THE LEG
WITH THE KNOBBLE II

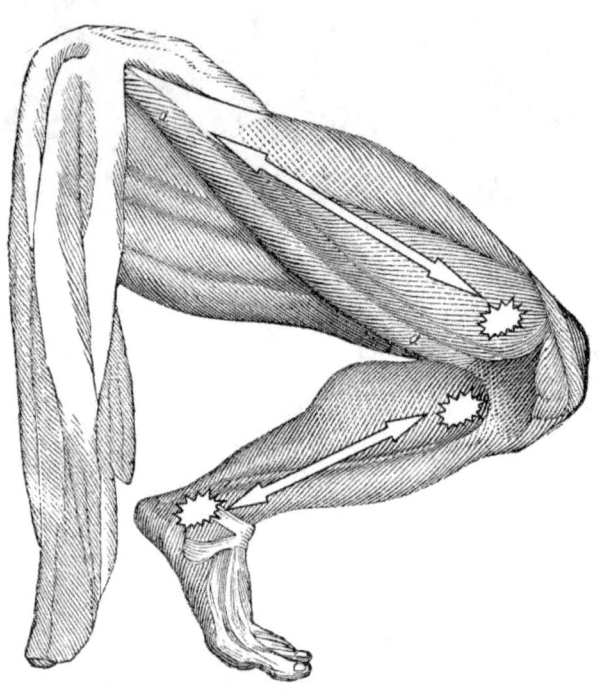

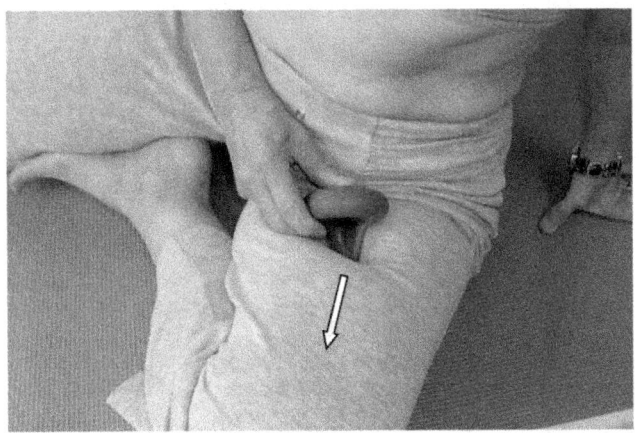

When you start applying pressure you can feel if you are in the right place. Work your way down to the knee.

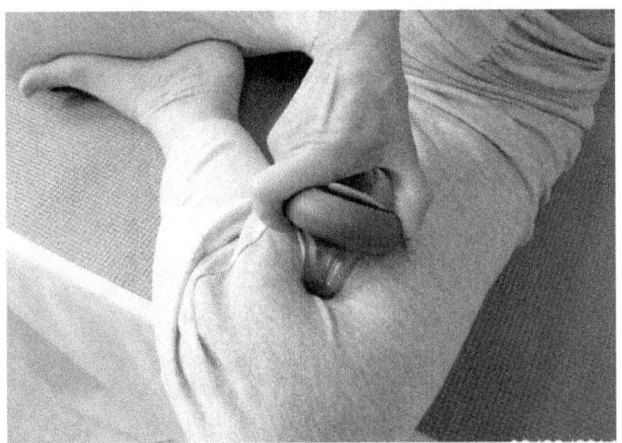

Working the area close to the knee can help knee pain.
Caution: *Never apply pressure to the knee cap itself*
Work the area around the knee only.

INSIDE THE LEG WITH THE FINGERS

The inside of your lower leg may be very sensitive.
Begin at the ankle and work your way up.

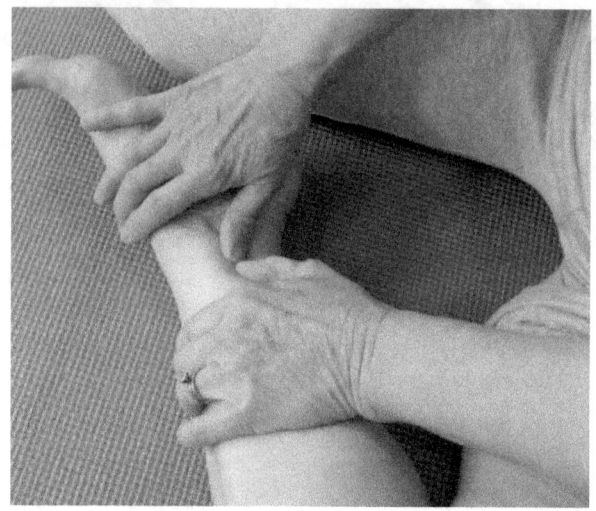

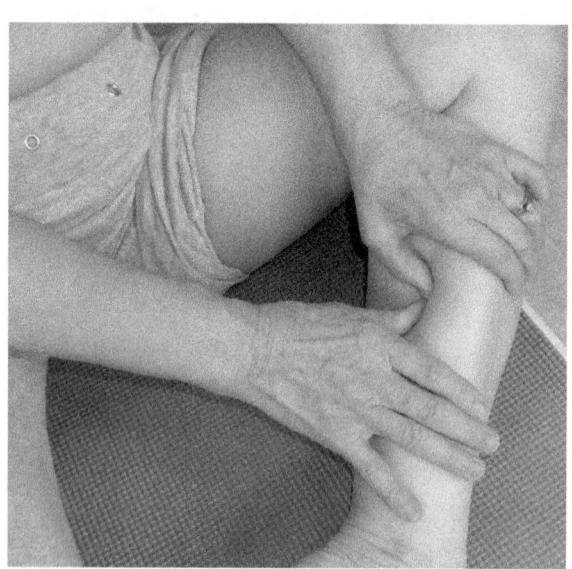

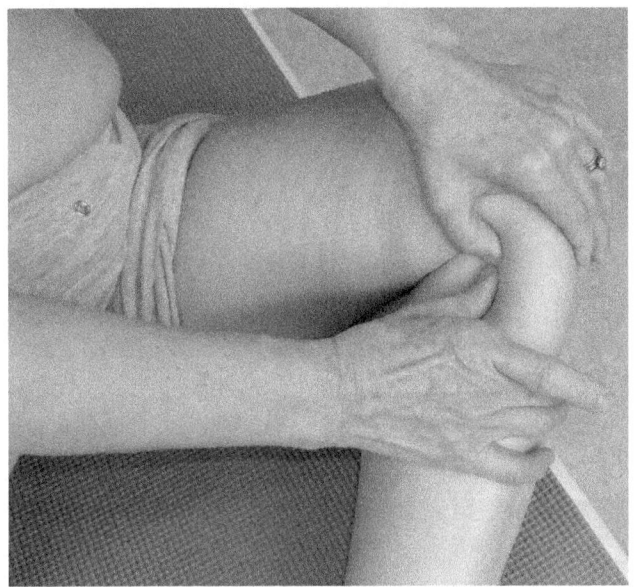

5 BODY ARCHING

Body Arching helps relieve sciatic nerve pain and low back pain by relieving the compression of the discs, compressing the overstretched muscles, and lengthening the shortened or compressed muscles. The pumping motion will increase blood and lymph flow, bringing in oxygen and nutrients. Increasing circulation will also help remove metabolic waste products and toxins.

There are 2 methods to accomplish this movement, the push up method and the ball method.
Either method is opening up the front of the vertebrae and relieving the compression of the sciatic nerve.

Follow Body Arching with an exercise in the opposite direction such as bending over to touch the toes. You can lie on the floor on your back and bring your knees to your chest.

Body Arching is important to do after prolonged sitting, bending over, or lifting heavy objects. If you are too tired to do either, roll up a towel and lie down with the towel under the curve of your back for 10-30 minutes. This will be even more effective if you also used a heating pad.

Check with you health care professional before beginning these exercises, if you have any of the following conditions:

1. Severe pain in the leg below the knee
2. Sensations of weakness, numbness, or pins and needles in your feet or toes
3. Your low back pain started after a recent severe accident.
4. After having severe low back pain, you develop bladder problems.

Body Arching may help you if:

Your pain is in the lower back,
 Your pain is brought on by prolonged sitting, bending over, or lifting heavy objects,
Even though walking or lying down may bring some relief of your pain, you cannot do either for very long,
You constantly need to alternate positions,
Bed rest requires that one or both legs must be propped up with a pillow,
You may have to get out of bed in the morning before you are ready, because you have to get up and walk,
You have lived with this pain for months or years and it is not getting any better,
Your health care professional has ruled out any health problems.

When beginning this program you will have temporary new pain and stiffness. You are exercising and pulling on muscles and soft tissues. This new pain can be worse than the pain you are trying to relieve. It will get better.

GOOD PAIN, BAD PAIN

The centralization of the pain is your main guide to continue this exercise, either the Push UP Method or the Body Rolling. When you pain moves from across the low back or from the buttock or thigh, to the center of your back, that is good.

If the pain moves away from the center of your back into one side of the buttock or thigh, stop this exercise. This could indicate that your herniated disc is pressing into the spinal column. Only a MRI can determine which direction your disc is pressing.

Cautions:

Check with your doctor before doing these exercises if you are over 60.

Do not do if your doctor has told you not to arch your back.

If you have had back surgery, do not do without your doctor's permission.

If you have a diagnosis of spinal stenosis or spondylolisthesis do not do these exercises.

If pain radiates into your legs while doing this exercise, stop.

If you have any condition with an abnormal spinal curvature or exaggerated lumbar arch, do not do this exercise.

MCKENZIE PUSH UP

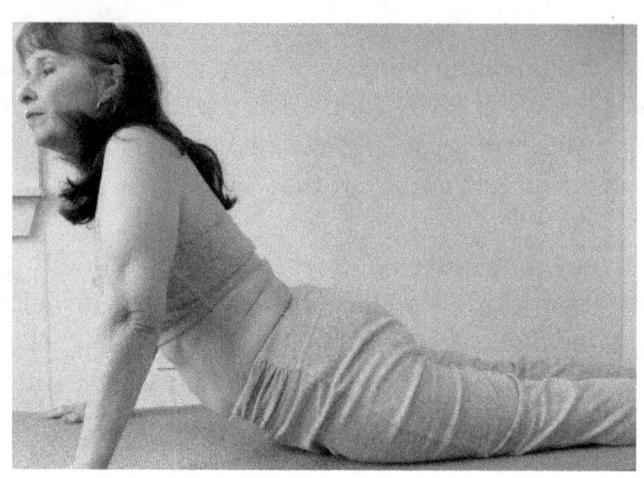

BODY ARCHING WITH A BALL

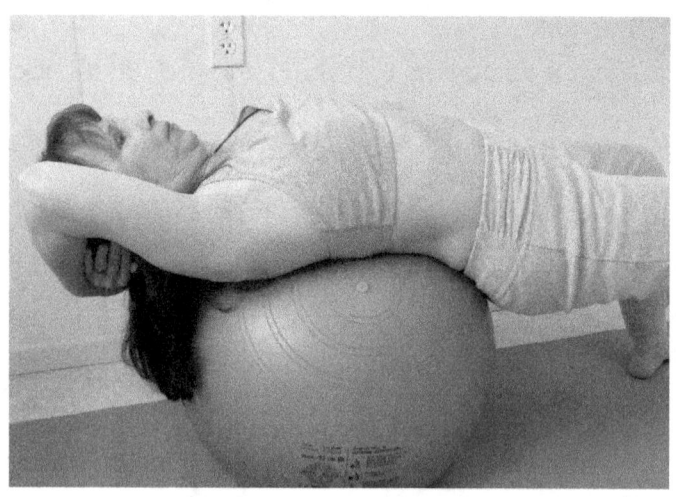

THE PUSH UP METHOD

The push up method was developed by Robin McKenzie. This is not for strengthening the back muscles. This push up is for relieving back pain. The sag in the low back is crucial to success.

Robin McKenzie of New Zealand established the McKenzie Institute International Spinal Therapy and Rehabilitation Centres to treat persons with chronic low back and neck pain. He promotes self-treatment as the long term solution to chronic pain. He has written 4 books and has developed the Original McKenzie Lumbar Rolls and Cervical Rolls. He has been instrumental in the redesign of furniture and car seats to provide lumbar support.

Treat Your Own Back by Robin McKenzie is a history of the McKenzie method with many illustrations for treatment and prevention of low back pain.

Place elbows under the shoulders and push up. Keep the pelvis, hips, and legs on the floor. Allow the low back to sag. Hold the sag position at least 1-2 seconds. If this is comfortable, hold for a longer period of time. Repeat 10 times if you are comfortable doing so.

Repeat at least 3 times a day the first few days. During the first few days the pain in your low back may be worse than the sciatic nerve pain. Your pain is centralizing.

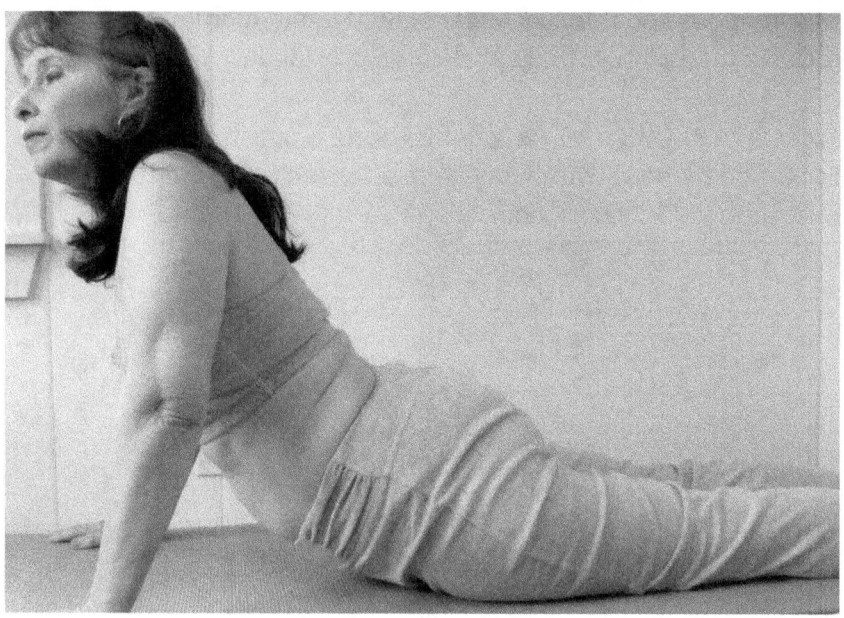

Once your original pain is under control and you are over the new pain and stiffness, repeat this exercise once in the morning and night.

If you are experiencing pain in one side of the body, lower the leg of the side of the body that is hurting

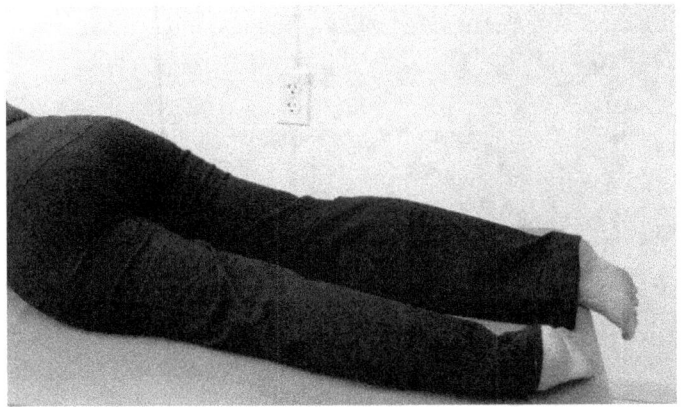

This is hard to demonstrate in a picture. You will understand when you see it in the class.

BODY ARCHING WITH A BALL

You can use the large exercise balls or the play balls.

When you are first suffering from sciatic nerve pain, you may have to repeat this exercise several times a day. Because the nerves are irritated, you may not think it is working until the next day.

Because this is an exercise you may be sore from stretching muscles you are not accustomed to working. It is especially important to do after you have been sitting or bending for long periods of time.

Caution: you can roll off the ball and injure yourself. Do not do if you have limited mobility.

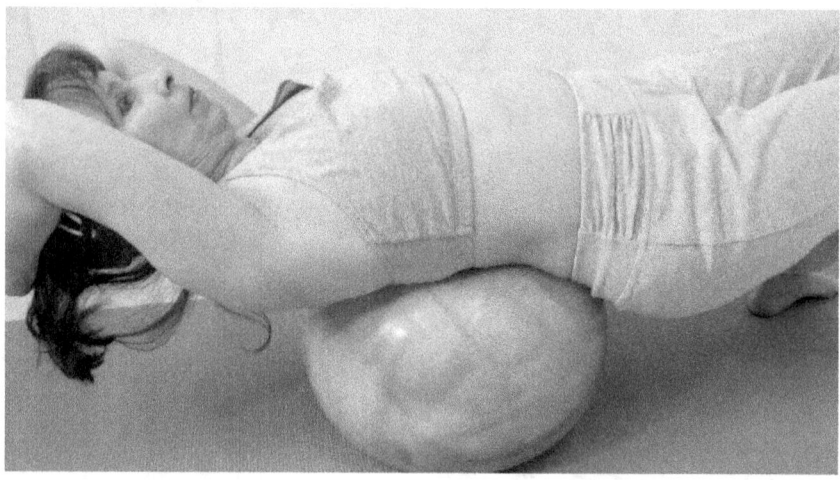

Any new exercise program will create some muscle stiffness and pain. To avoid pain, do one set of Body Arching with Ball or the Push Up every other day and work up to 3 times a day to relieve your low pain or sciatic nerve pain. You may not experience relief as quickly but you will avoid the muscle pain and soreness.

Squat in front of the ball. Get your balance. Knees bent and legs spread apart.

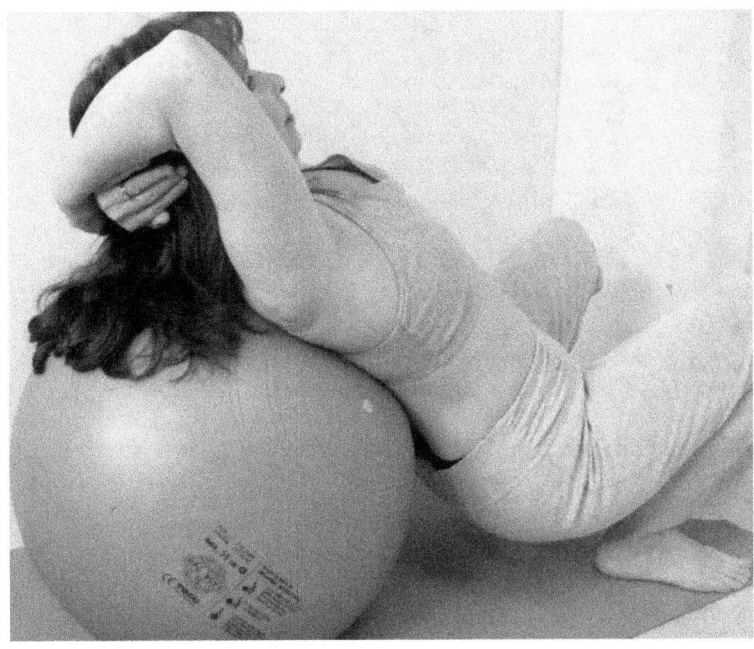

Give yourself a push.

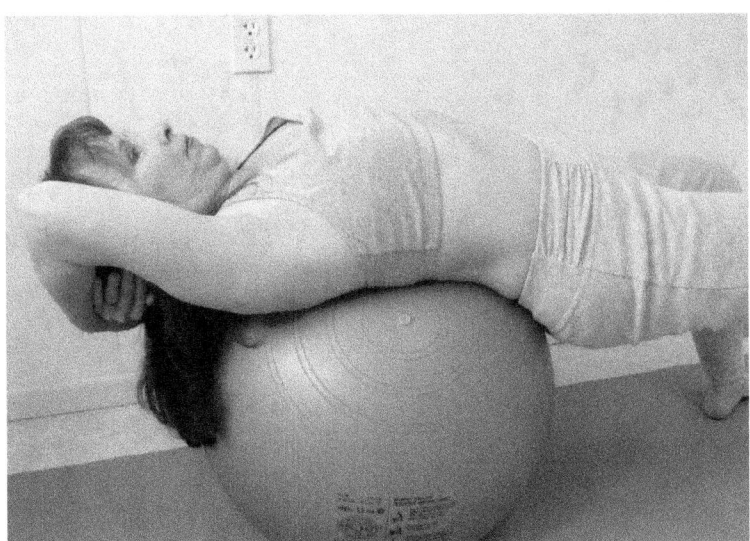

Roll all the way back and hold for a count of 8 seconds.

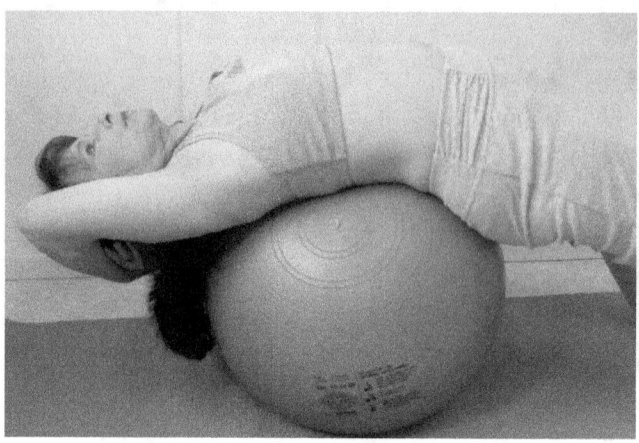

Come back to your beginning position and repeat 8 times.

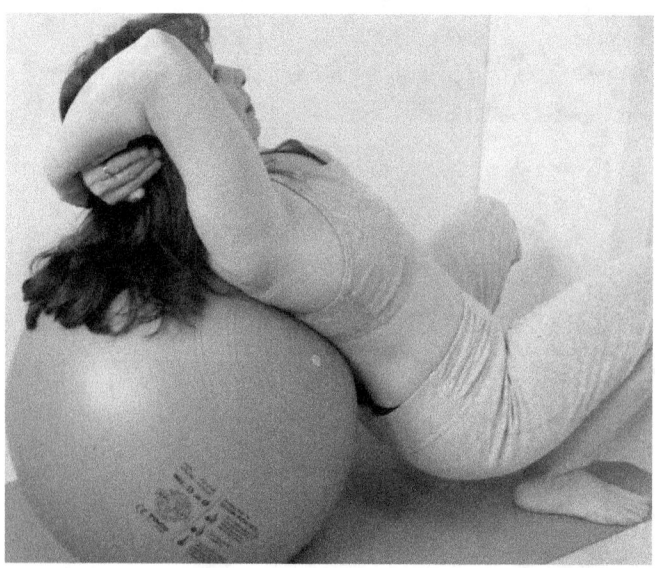

Your goal is the arching of the back to open up the front of your spinal column.

Depending on your fitness level, lying in the beginning position for 10 seconds may be all you need to do.

6 BODY ROLLING

Trigger Point is all about relaxing the muscles and releasing constriction in the muscles.

Stretching or elongating the muscles, give these constrictions somewhere to go and help to re- educate the muscle.

When massaging our clients we may use effleurage, gliding strokes and stretches to accomplish this purpose.

In this class we are using Body Rolling. My reference for this body work is this book, Body Rolling by Yamuna Zake and Stephanie Golden. This body work is based on yoga.

I have had no training in Yoga. I use this body work for self treatment of a combination of light Trigger Point and stretching the muscles. You might say this is a gentler, softer form of Trigger Point.

I am not teaching yoga, but I am using the same principal for stretching and elongating the muscles.

We have 2 sizes of balls here. If you are under 5 4", choose the 6"-8" ball and if you are taller, choose the 9"-10" ball.

These are inexpensive vinyl play balls that are hollow. I bought them at the Dollar Store. You can get more expensive inflatable balls at the sporting goods store or sporting goods department of bigger stores.
The less air the balls have in them, the better you can balance on them, and the softer they will feel to your body.

If you get more into this, purchase the professional balls and this book, Body Rolling.

This will require 15 - 20 minutes.

Use this time as a self help and as you feel the benefits think about gliding up or down your client's back.

According to the Yoga philosophy your healing energy is located at the base of the spine. I believe it is all about the pelvis being your center of balance.

We will begin body rolling at the (1) Ischium or sitz bones, roll to (2) the Coccyx, roll up (3) the Sacrum, (4) the pelvic or Iliac crest, and roll on up the spine. As you roll up the spine you are creating space between the vertebrae, elongating the spinal muscles. And according to Yoga, so that your healing energy can move freely.

You always work both sides of the spine.

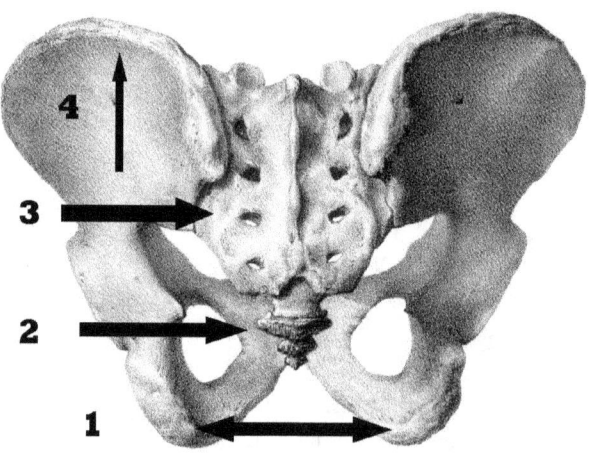

We will start out getting comfortable on the ball.

There is no absolute correct way to do this. Do what is comfortable for you. Have fun. You do not look any sillier than your neighbor.

Remember to breathe and sink into the ball.

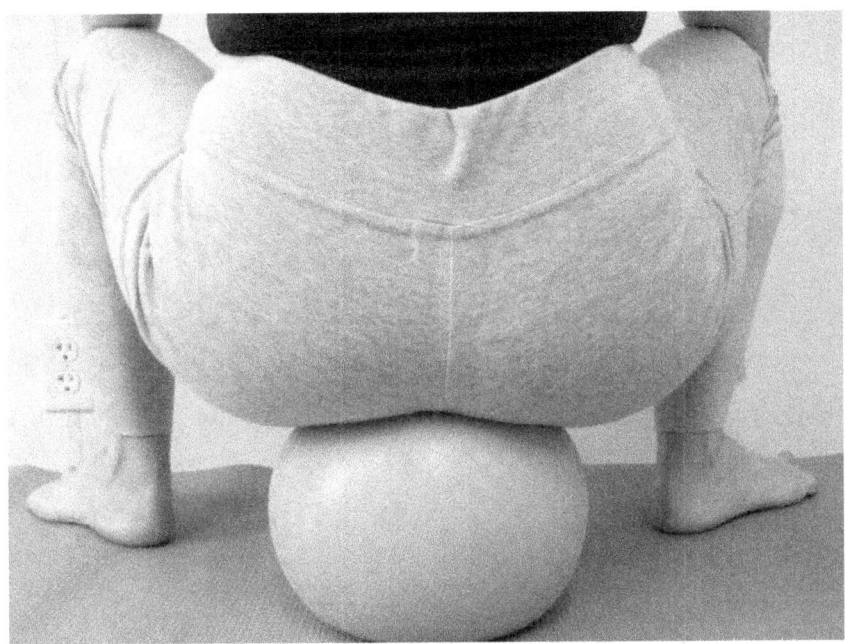

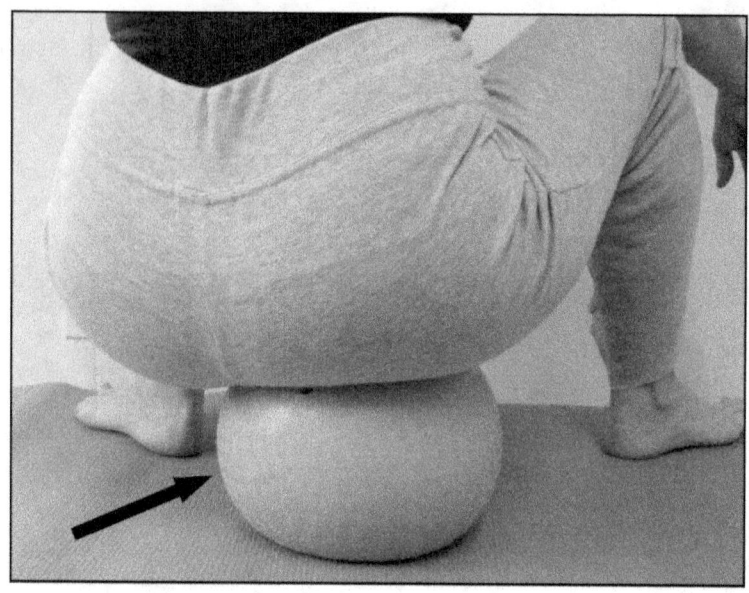

Roll downwards on the right side angling into the Ischium (1) or sitz bone and roll around.

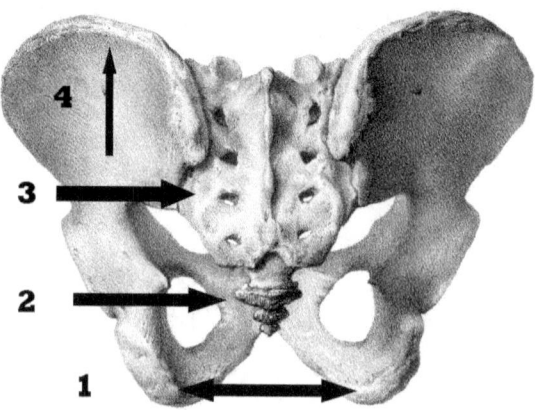

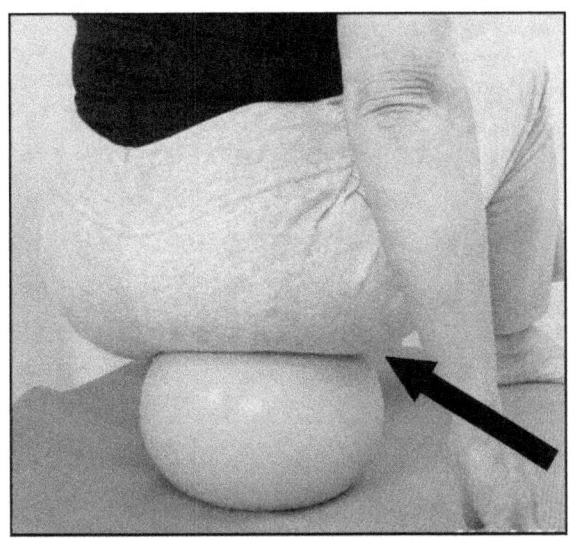

Roll up angling into the coccyx (2) and the sacrum (3).

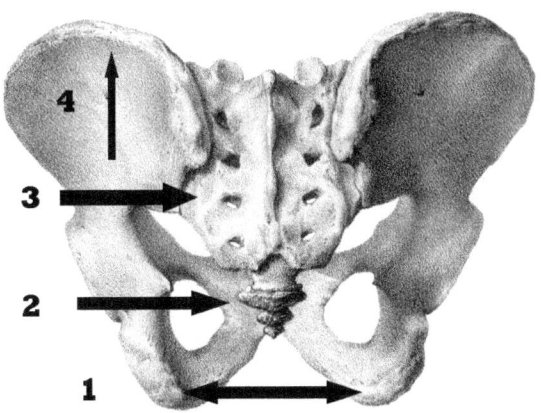

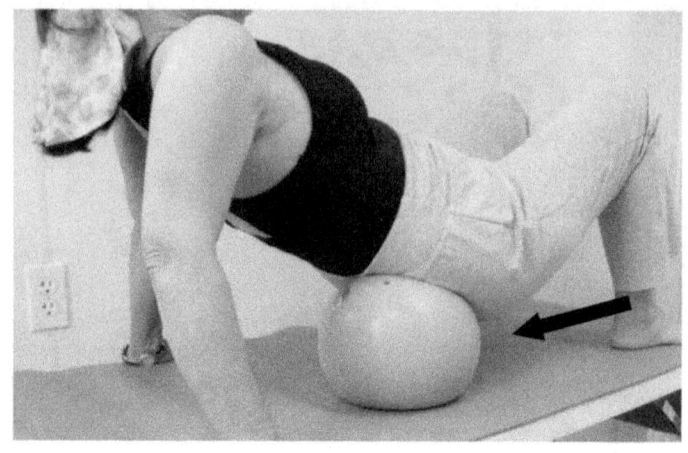

Roll up to the Iliac Crest (4)

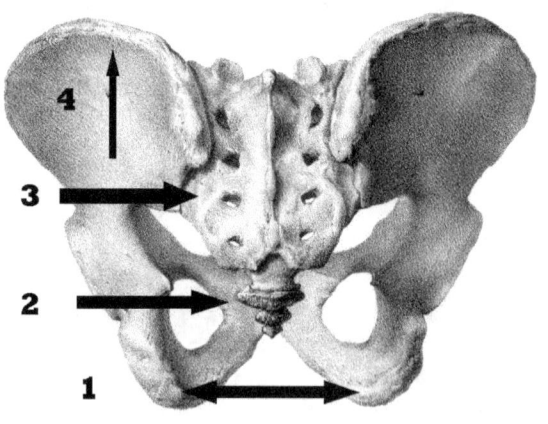

Roll back up to the spine, and then continue rolling up the right side of the spine to the shoulder.

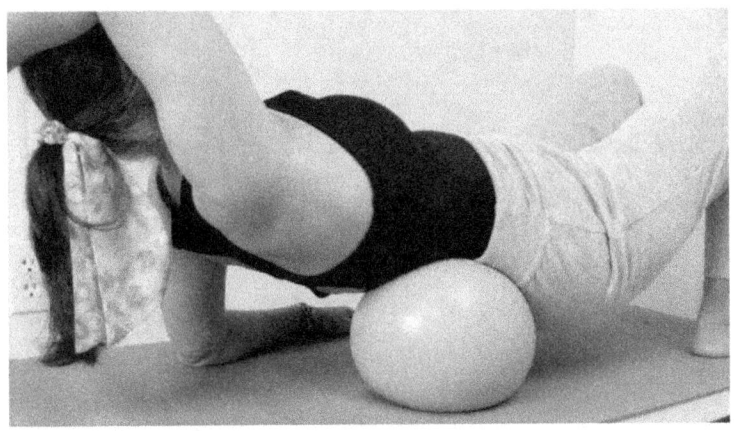

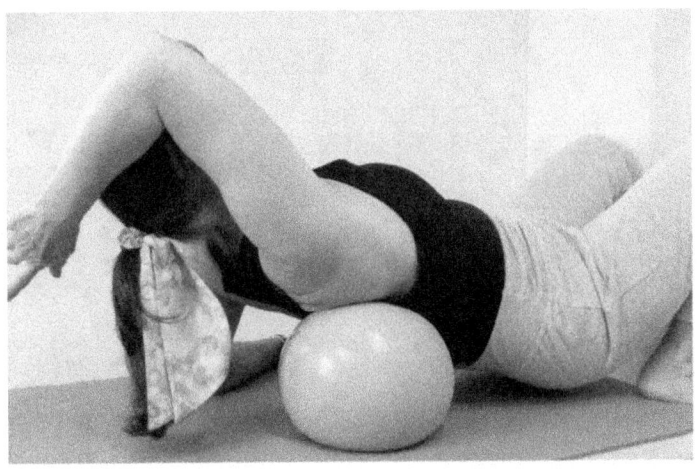

When you get to the neck, roll across the shoulder and then come back to the neck.

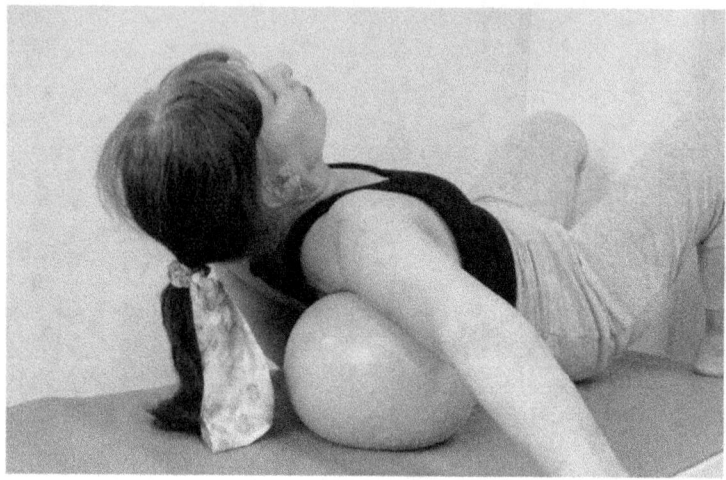

Go up the neck.

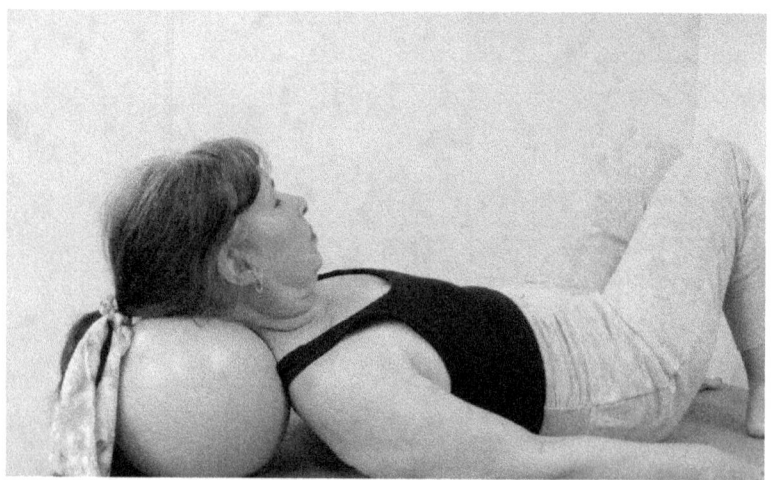

After resting at the neck, turn head and rest.

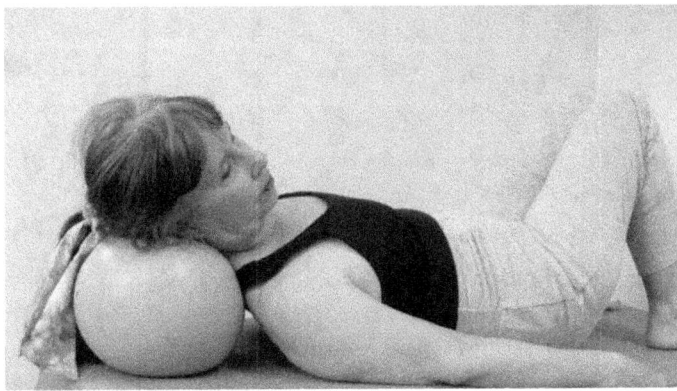

You will now need to pick up your ball and go back to your starting place on the floor and repeat the process on the opposite side of the body.

After you have done the opposite side of the body, come back and sit on your ball and then roll up the center of your spine.

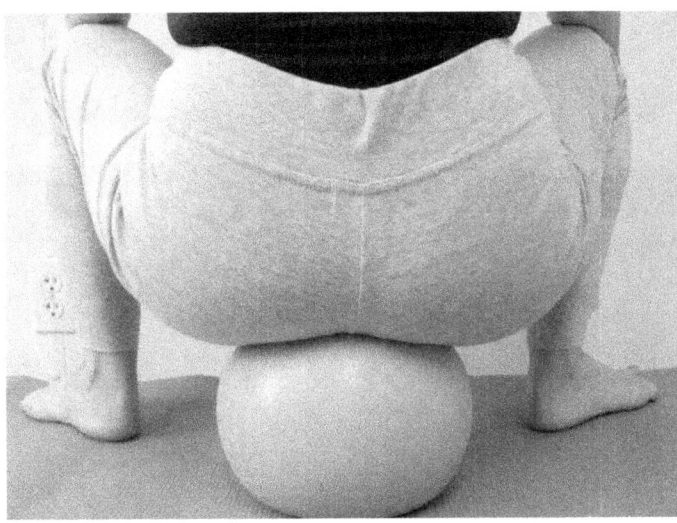

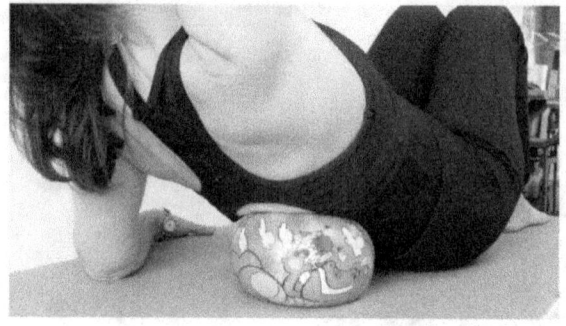

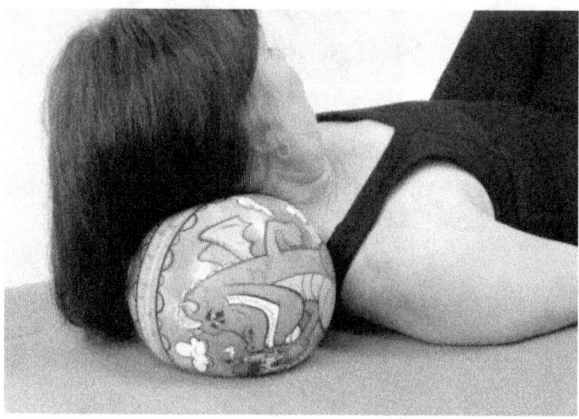

Rolling up the spine will help with sciatica if there is pressure on the sciatic nerve in the lumbar.

Lie there and breathe.

Everyone get up and walk around for about 5 minutes.

Do you feel taller? Are you breathing deeper?

Does your back feel straighter?

FRONT ON THE NECK AND CHEST WITH BALL

The sternum or chest bone has many Trigger Points. Muscles attach here that can pull your neck and shoulders down and forward. These Trigger Points may also prevent you from being able to breathe deeply.

Making sounds and deep coughing while doing this bodywork may help release repressed emotions held in the chest and diaphragm similar to Reichian emotional release work.

Giving your clients permission to moan and groan during a massage will also help them release stress.

You may be very tender here and need to support yourself with your arms.

Caution: Do not do if you have had open heart surgery or have broken your chest bone.

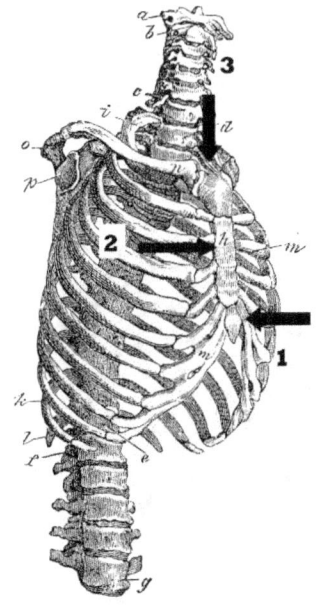

3. Clavicles

2. Sternum

1. Xiphoid Process

Lie on the ball above the Xiphoid Process. Relax and breathe for 30 seconds. Your are pushing the ball into the sternum. You are beginning to relax the muscles of the neck, shoulders and the chest.

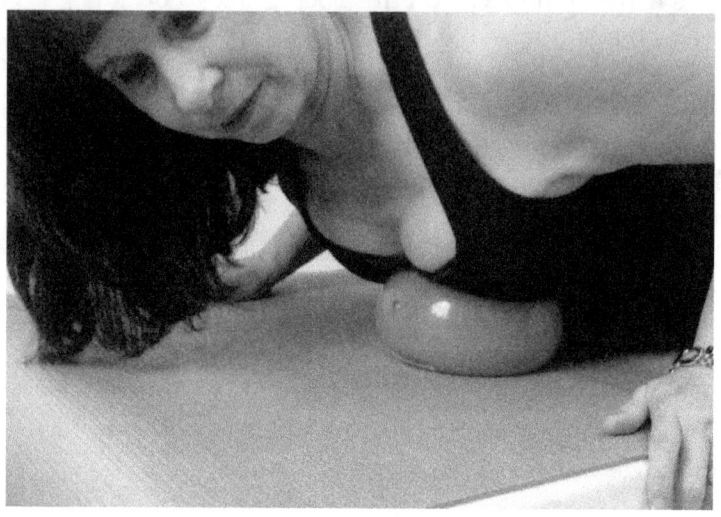

Roll the ball halfway up the sternum. Relax and breathe 30 seconds.

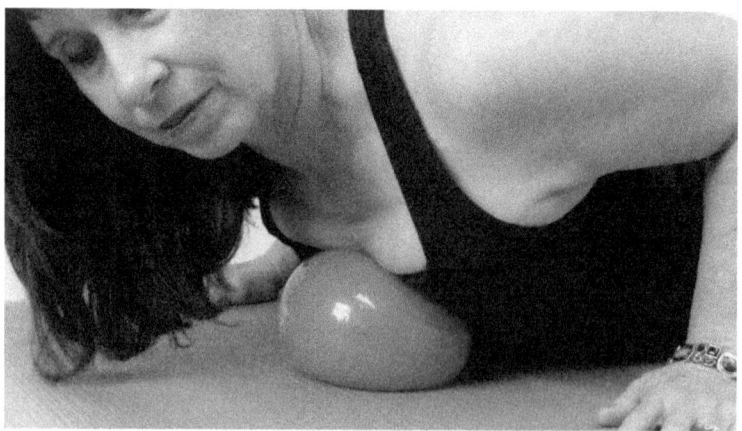

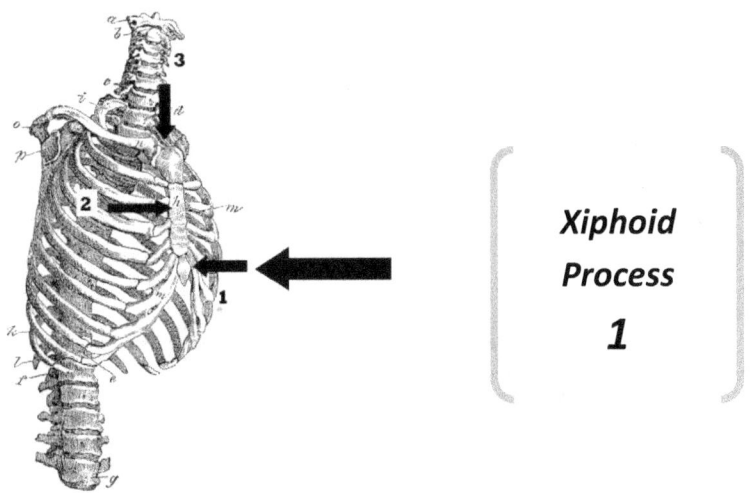

Xiphoid
Process
1

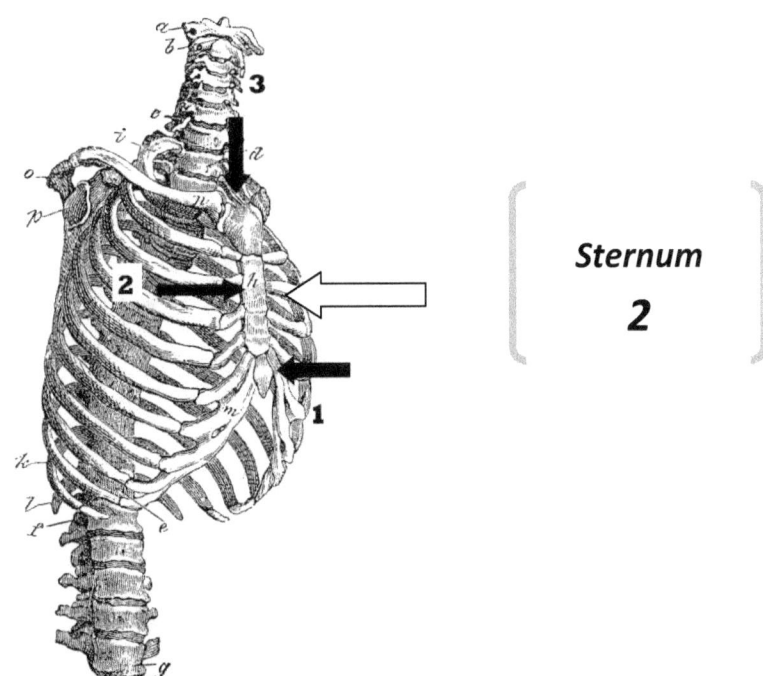

Sternum

2

Roll the ball up to where the clavicles meet. Relax and breathe 30 seconds.

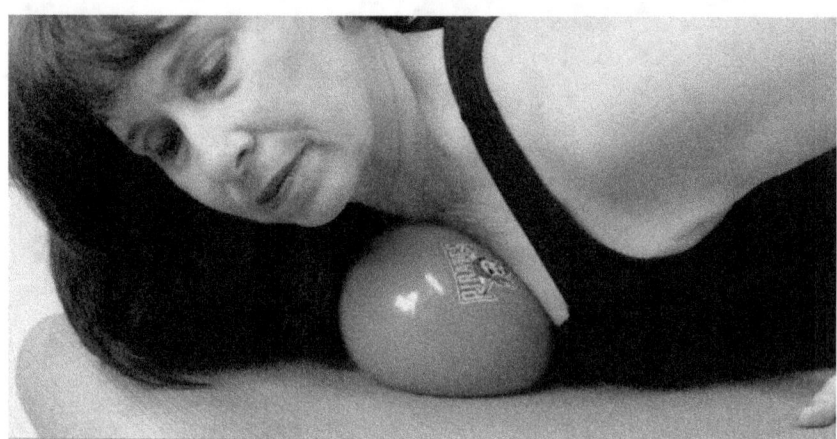

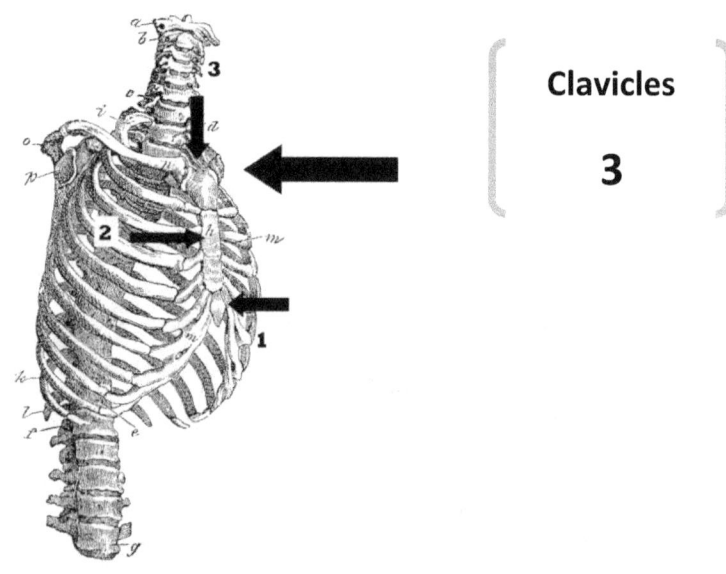

Clavicles

3

These exercises have helped me learn to deep breathe. Until I released these muscles I really could not take a deep breath.

I have always been a shallow breather. My husband is a smoker and I am not. When we did a breathing test, the respiratory therapist thought I was the smoker and my husband the non-smoker. I thought it was because I was born with under developed lungs. I had tried and tried deep breathing techniques including self-hypnosis. I just could not get my breath to go into my belly. After doing these exercises I can now deep breathe.

This exercise has also corrected my bad habit of walking with my head down. I assure you I would have never stepped on a snake because I always walked looking down. I thought it was because I was nearsighted.

 NO, it was those tight muscles pulling my head down. I now walk looking up, enjoying nature in a new way.

Of course, I now stand the possibility of stepping on a snake!

While we have the ball, we might as well treat these areas while we are here.

1.The Pecs, causes rounded shoulders and pain in chest area, including down the arm, inside the forearm and down to the 4th and 5th fingers.

2.Treat the Latissimus Dorsi, which may also cause pain under the scapula and go down the arm into the 4th and 5th fingers.

3.Subscapularis,may cause pain at top of shoulder, under arm, and wrist, unable to go across to opposite arm pit.

4.Serratus Anterior, may cause chest pain, shortness of breath, and pain down the arm to 4th and 5th
fingers.

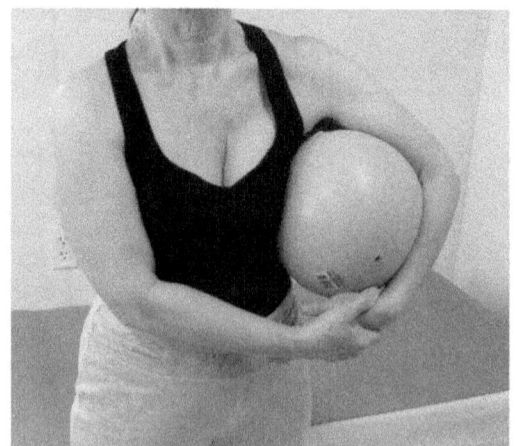

Applying pressure beside the breast and under the arm to get to the Latissimus Dorsi, Subscapularis, and the Serratus Anterior.

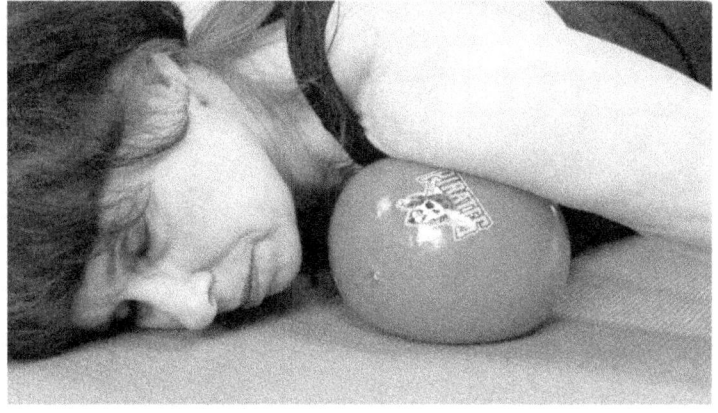

Apply pressure with a ball to treat the pecs.

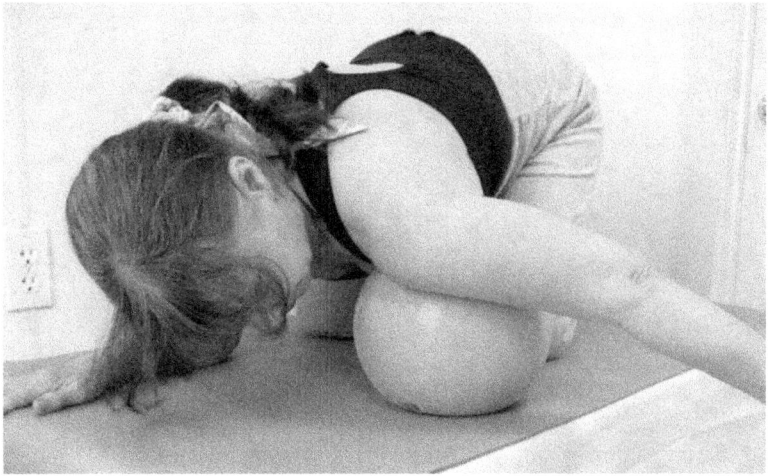

Deeper pressure with a ball.

7 DEEP BREATHING

Research shows deep breathing to be the single most effective medicine to treat stress. Deep breathing slows the heart rate, decreases blood pressure, relaxes the muscles and calms the mind, decreasing anxiety. Deep breathing helps your muscles elongate. Deep breathing at bedtime signals your body to relax.

Are you breathing correctly? Are you a shallow breather? Deep breathing doesn't work if you are not doing it correctly.

As a baby you started out breathing naturally. When you breathed in, your belly stuck out because your diaphragm was drawing in air. When you breathed out, your belly sucked in because your diaphragm was pushing out the air. Are you now breathing just the opposite?

What happened?

It may have started as a defense mechanism. We were yelled out as kids, maybe we were overly sensitive or physically or mentally abused and we tighten the rib cage in defense. After all, one of the functions of the ribs is to protect the heart and the lungs.

It may have started with health problems.

Self Image, women may tighten up the chest area trying to look smaller and thinner for today's fashion.
Men may tighten up the chest area for that Napoleon or muscle man posture.

We are taught to suck in our guts and stick out our chest. Everyone stand up. Head held high, chest stuck out, belly in. Really? Can you breathe correctly in that position?

Contracted muscles in the chest are related to chronic neck and shoulder tension. They can also be the cause of headaches.

In my practice it has been my experience that shallow breathers experience the most problems with chronic pain and tension. Contracted, tense muscles produce pain, fatigue, and lowers your immune system.

My husband is a deep breather. The only time he hurts is when he has actually injured himself or had over done physical work.

Even though I know all about deep breathing, it is a constant job for me to remember to breathe deep.

Shallow breathers hurt because they simply wake up each morning.

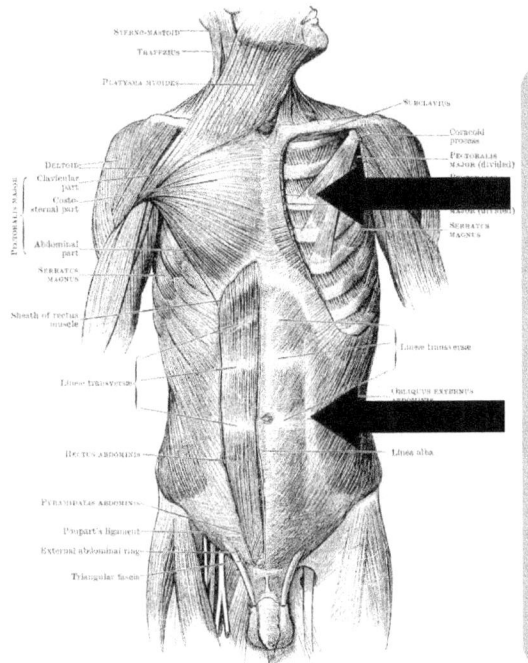

Shallow breathers use top part of lungs. Fight or Flight Response

Deep breathers breathe all the way down. A-OK Relax

Shallow breathers are using only the top part of their lungs.

Breathing at the top part of your lungs signals your body's fight or flight response, the sympathetic nervous system.

It is telling your body to tense up and be ready for action.

It is physically impossible to fully relax if you are breathing with the top part of your lungs.

Deep breathers breathe all the way down to their belly. Breathing all the way down into your belly, signals your body's relaxation response, the parasympathetic nervous system.

Your brain is getting the message that everything is A-OK, go ahead and relax.

Full natural breathing uses both the chest and the belly.

Lie down.
Place the ball on your belly.
Inhale. 1-2-3-4-5
Exhale. 1-2-3-4-5

Did you belly come up when you inhaled or did it go down?
If your belly sucked in when you inhaled, you are a shallow breather.

If your belly raised the ball up when you inhaled, congratulations, you are breathing correctly.

Let's all breathe correctly.

Place the ball on your belly.
Inhale, as you breathe in try to push the ball up with your belly. 1-2-3-4-5
Exhale, as you breathe out, let the ball fall into your belly.1-2-3-4-5

8 GLIDING OR EFFLEURAGE

My experience in receiving massage therapy is that the Massage Therapist has gotten so caught up in advanced techniques that he or she has forgotten the basics of massage which is to first relax the client.

I have gotten very little effleurage or gliding strokes at the beginning of the massage. The therapist doesn't go beyond spreading the lotion.

Superficial gliding not only spreads the lotion, but accustoms the client to the therapist touch.

It produces a soothing effect.

It allows the therapist to assess the body area being massaged.

It is especially beneficial to do between deeper or intense work to clear and soothe the area that has just been worked.

Think about when you go to a club, listen to music on the radio, or when they play music at church. They alternate slow music with fast music. A good movie relieves the intense moments with laughter or some tender moments.

A good massage will also alternate intense work with light work. Deep work is cleared and soothed with effleurage.

Deep gliding or effleurage stretches and broadens the muscle and fascia. When Trigger Points are released they need somewhere to go. Muscles will be re-educated to relax through the stretching or deep gliding.

9 ANTI-INFLAMMATORIES

Unlike many advanced techniques which claim to be the cure for everything, I do not make that claim.

Trigger Point Therapy will bring relief from pain caused by muscle tension.
It does not relieve inflammation. It may release tensed muscles that may be causing the inflammation.
It will not relieve joint inflammation. It will not relieve pain and soreness from overworked muscles or even the pain and soreness that come from doing this bodywork.

As you learn to release muscle tension, you will then learn to recognize which pain is tension and which pain what may be joint inflammation. You will learn which pain may just be muscle soreness.

Yes you may need to use some anti- inflammatories. Aspirin and Ibuprofen are anti-inflammatories. Tylenol, though a pain reliever is not an anti-inflammatory. Using them occasionally may be alright. They do come with their risks.

When one of my client's wife died from overuse of Tylenol, I got real serious about finding a natural anti-inflammatory.

One natural anti-inflammatory is an extract from hops. Hops is an herb used to give beer a pleasant bitter flavor.

15 years of research has proven hops extract to be an effective pain reliever without the adverse effects of NSAIDS.

All hops extracts are not equal. The powder form is the easiest to find. I have concluded from my research that the liquid extract of hops is much more effective.

Vinoprin is a liquid extract of hops. So far I have not found any other brands that are a liquid.

www.vinoprin

Turmeric and Ginger are natural anti-inflammatories.

I take Osteo Bi-Flex a glucosamine supplement for my joints. It has 5-Loxin Advanced for joint comfort. 5-Loxin Advanced is Boswellia Serrata extract, otherwise known as Frankincense.

Stressed out nerves will cause inflammation. B vitamins are good for nerves.

Calcium makes muscles contract, magnesium causes muscles to relax. Magnesium is called the calming mineral.

Remember why people take Milk of Magnesia. When taking a magnesium supplement, begin with the lowest dose recommended or even half as much and work your way up to more.

Dehydration causes muscle contractions. The fluid between our vertebrae and joints require water.

10 TIPS FOR INTEGRATING TRIGGER POINT THERAPY INTO A RELAXING MASSAGE

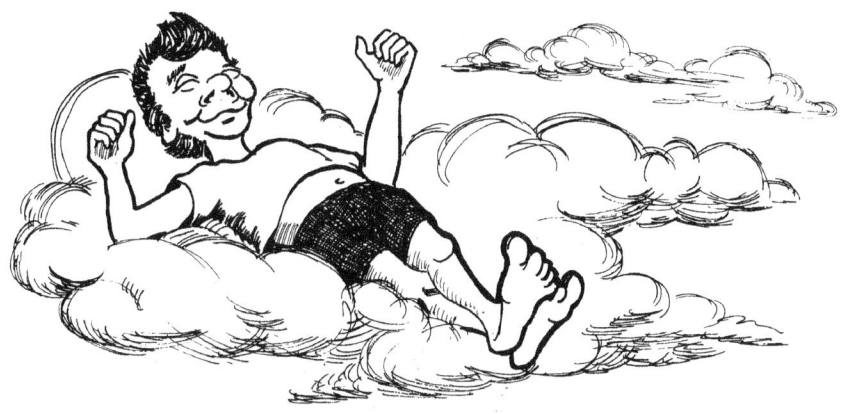

Generally speaking , new clients are not looking for physical therapy, they are not looking for a chiropractor, nor do they want an exercise coach. They want to relax and they want their pain to go away with no work or effort on their part. They really don't even want you asking too many questions.

How is this nearly impossible mission accomplished?

When your client is filling out the client information sheet (required by law) explain to them about Trigger Point. Remember all clients will not enjoy Trigger Point nor benefit from Trigger Point. Although once you start practicing Trigger Point you will find that you will draw clients that need Trigger Point to you and your clients will be recommending their friends and relatives.

It is pretty easy to press a Trigger Point on their shoulder and explain to them that the pressure should be "oh that hurts so good" or "stop don't do that, that hurts."

Explain to them it is not a pain endurance contest, and taking more pressure than is comfortable does not make it work any better.

Explain to them that you do not know how much pressure they can take unless they communicate to you that the pressure is either too much or not enough.

Explain to them about deep breathing and breathing into the pain.

You will not start your therapy with Trigger Point. You will not apply Trigger Point all over their body at once. You will start with effleurage or deep gliding and integrate Trigger Point into the massage.

You will integrate this into your massage using your own techniques. This is just an example how I do it.

Demonstrated in class.

ABOUT THE AUTHOR

Carolyn Gibson has been a Licensed Massage Therapist since 1996. She practices her profession at their farm, Dogwood Gardens Organic Farm in Ben Wheeler TX 75754.

Carolyn first experienced the effectiveness of massage on her husband disabled in the Vietnam war. She knew nothing then of massage, she just had her natural instincts to guide her.

After graduating from Hands on Therapy in Garland Texas and taking other CE classes she still suffered chronic headaches and pain and tension in the shoulders and neck.

She lived out on the farm and had no other fellow massage therapists to trade massages with or to practice on.

A massage instructor recommended Pain Erasure by Bonnie Prudden. She was determined to end her pain and tension.

Bonnie's book was not written for self treatment. After discovering body tools she was able to use the information from Bonnie's book to learn Trigger Point and experience the relief of Trigger Point Therapy.

She used this knowledge to work on her many clients who came to her for pain and tension relief. Her clients were amazed when a simple country massage therapist was able to relieve their pain when the doctors, chiropractors, physical therapists and even other massage therapists were unable to help them.

Feedback from her clients and her own self treatment has taught her more than the many other Trigger Point classes she has taken.